Edward Jenner and Vaccination

Frontispiece Trying to trace the course of an outbreak of smallpox in Ethiopia: a health worker tries to find out the contacts this boy has had, before and after he caught the disease.

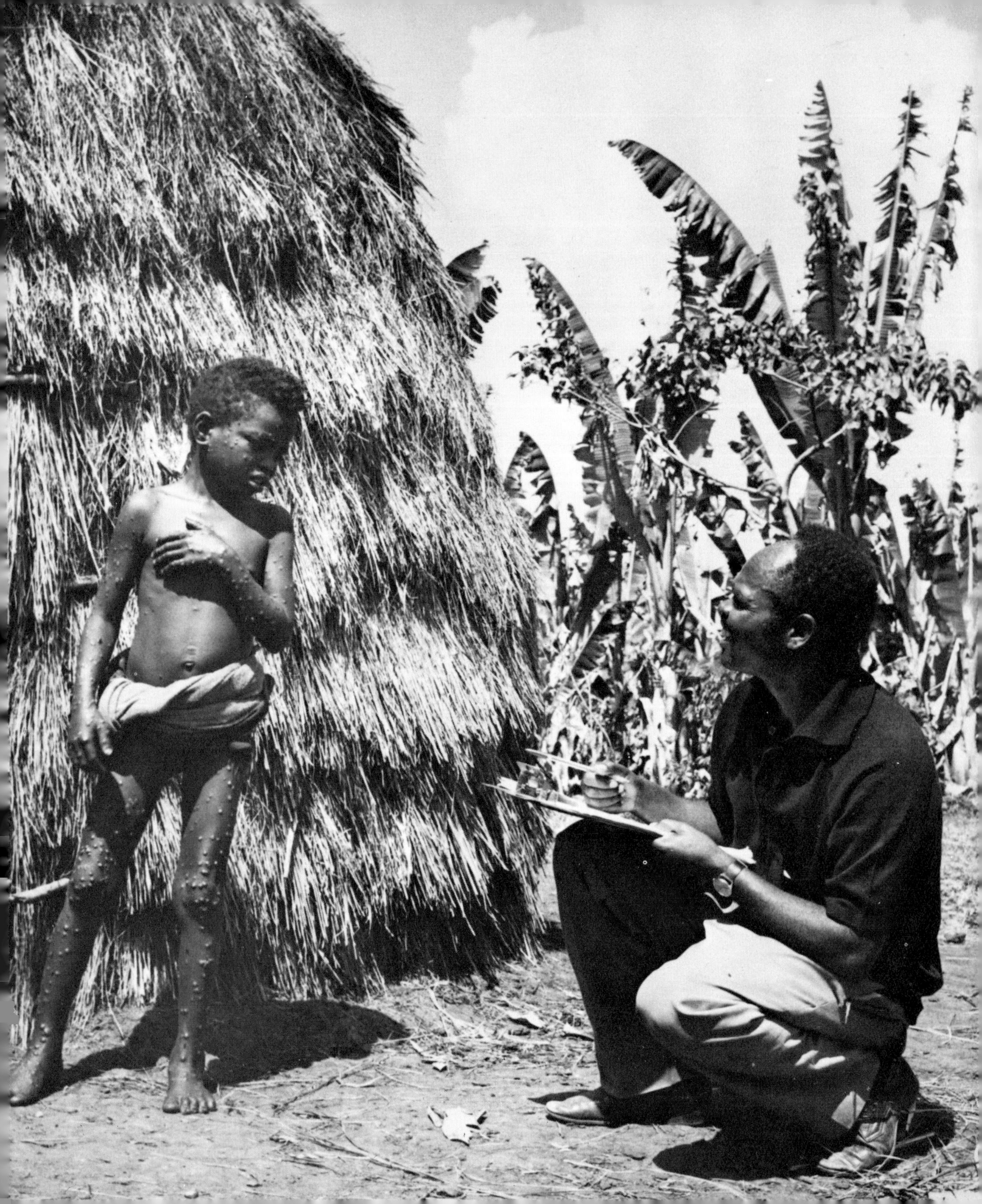

Pioneers of Science and Discovery

Edward Jenner
and Vaccination

A. J. Harding Rains M.S., F.R.C.S.

Professor of Surgery
Charing Cross Hospital Medical School,
University of London

Honorary Consultant Surgeon
Charing Cross Hospital

Member of Council
Royal College of Surgeons of England

PRIORY PRESS LIMITED

Other Books in this Series

Carl Benz and the Motor Car Doug Nye
George Eastman and the Early Photographers Brian Coe
Alexander Fleming and Penicillin W Howard Hughes
Richard Arkwright and Cotton Spinning Richard L Hills
Joseph Lister and Antisepsis William Merrington
Edward Jenner and Vaccination A J Harding Rains
James Simpson and Chloroform R S Atkinson
Louis Pasteur and Microbiology H I Winner
Alfred Nobel, Inventor of Explosives Trevor I Williams
William Harvey and Blood Circulation Eric Neil
Isaac Newton and Gravity P M Rattansi
Rudolph Diesel and the Power Unit John F Moon
Michael Faraday and Electricity Brian Bowers

SBN 85078 118 3

First published in 1974 by
Priory Press Ltd, 101 Grays Inn Road, London, W.C.1.
Set in 'Monophoto' Baskerville and printed offset litho by
Page Bros (Norwich) Ltd, Norwich

Contents

Vaccination—an Introduction
1 Jenner's Life
2 Jenner's World
3 Jenner and Hunter
4 The Natural Historian
5 Smallpox
6 Cow Pox and Vaccination
7 Vaccination Grows in Britain
8 World Opinion, Past and Present
Date Chart
Glossary
Further Reading
Index

List of Illustrations

Tracing smallpox contacts in Ethiopia *frontispiece*
Edward Jenner 8
Decline in world smallpox outbreaks 9
Smallpox in Ancient Egypt 9
Scenes of Jenner's life 10
John Hunter 11
Catherine, Jenner's wife 12
Initials of Jenner's children 13
Berkeley Castle 16–17
Bone from a whale Jenner dissected 18
The Chantry, Berkeley 20
The Temple of Vaccinia 21
Robert Clive 22
Letter from Hunter to Jenner 22
An Inquiry into Cow Pox, title-page 23
Henry Cavendish, discoverer of hydrogen 25
Humphry Davey, discoverer of nitrous oxide 26
William Hunter 28
John Hunter's house at Earl's Court, London 29
Cuckoo's egg in the nest of another bird 35
Young cuckoo in lesser whitethroat's nest 36
Newly hatched cuckoo pushing egg out of nest 37
Two types of vaccinia 40
Child with smallpox 42–43
Arms and legs of smallpox sufferer 44
Scars left by smallpox 46–47
Map showing spread of smallpox across the world 48–49
Queen Mary of England 50
Early methods of fighting smallpox 51
Lady Mary Wortley Montagu 52
Dr. John Lettsom, supporter of Jenner 56
Medical instrument belonging to Jenner 56
Drawings of cow pox and smallpox made by Jenner 58–59

Jenner inoculates James Phipps 61
Jenner's letter to Gardner 63
Satire of Jenner's ideas 66–67
Cartoon against vaccination for smallpox 69
Vaccination became quite popular in time 72–73
Napoleon Bonaparte 76
President John Adams of America 78
Thomas Jefferson, President of America 80
Smallpox eradication campaign in Nepal 81
Queueing for vaccination in England 81
Floating smallpox hospitals on the Thames 82
Checking eradication programme in Ethiopia 83
How modern travel makes spreading smallpox easy 83
Modern vaccination methods 84
Manufacturing lymph for vaccine 85
The finished anti-smallpox vaccine 86–87

My thanks are due to the Royal College of Surgeons of England and the Royal College of Physicians for their library facilities.

I would also like to acknowledge the stimulus which followed visits to Berkeley and especially that given by Canon the Reverend and Mrs Gethyn-Jones of Berkeley. Special thanks are due to my wife, Mary, and my secretary, Miss Judith Bowdage, for their assistance in preparing and typing the manuscript.

Vaccination—an Introduction

Vaccination protects us from an acute infectious disease called smallpox. This immunity is achieved by the doctor putting into a healthy person a little of the virus of cow pox taken from the skin of infected calves, and known as calflymph.

Few diseases have been so destructive to human life as smallpox, also called Variola. The earliest accounts of its ravages are from the sixth century, when epidemics broke out in Arabia and Egypt. In the Middle Ages, the disease spread all through Europe. Smallpox has been known—and regarded with horror—in England since the thirteenth century, when it is thought to have been introduced by crusaders returning from the Middle East. Though it is rare today, two people died from this disfiguring disease in London in 1973 as a result of a laboratory "leak" of pox virus.

It was to a Gloucestershire-born surgeon, Edward Jenner, that the idea of protection by vaccination first occurred, towards the end of the eighteenth century.

Dr Jenner knew the popular country belief that persons who fell ill from cow pox became immune from the dreaded smallpox. Jenner reasoned that if he could deliberately transmit cow pox virus from one person to another by arm-to-arm inoculation then the result would be both a source of pox lymph, independent of the existence or otherwise of the natural disease in cows, and protection for those inoculated with the vaccine. Inoculation means introducing into the body certain products of disease through the skin of a healthy person, so giving "built-in" resistance to the disease.

In 1798, Jenner tried to start a system of vaccina-

Edward Jenner, whose work did so much to control the scourge of smallpox.

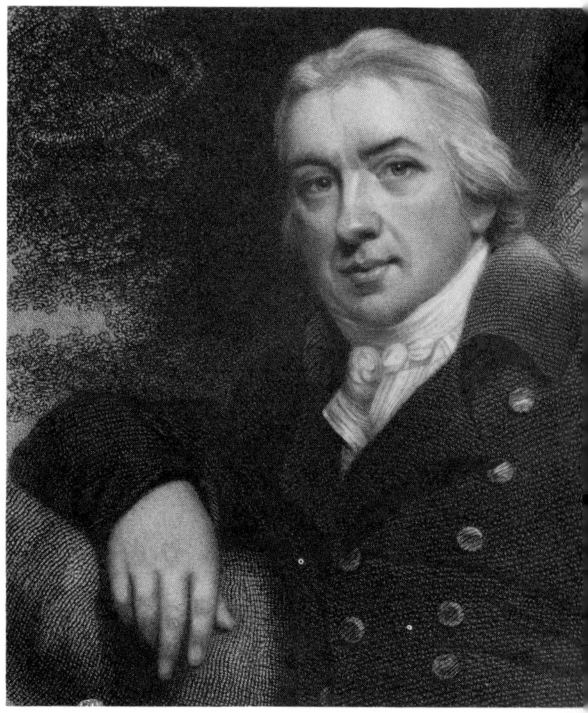

tion in London, but met with disbelief and angry opposition. Even so, he won a hearing from many influential people—including the Royal Family—and by 1853 vaccination was made compulsory in England, a situation which lasted until 1948. By this time, smallpox had become so rare in this country that vaccination became a voluntary (but still wise) precaution.

Jenner was truly one of the world's great medical benefactors. His work on vaccination laid the foundations for all modern immunological means of controlling diseases.

More than 200 years after his birth, we are today on the eve of the finest possible tribute to Jenner's life and work—the World Health Organization believes the last case of smallpox *anywhere in the world* will occur in 1974, and if these hopes are realized the scourge can be eradicated for ever.

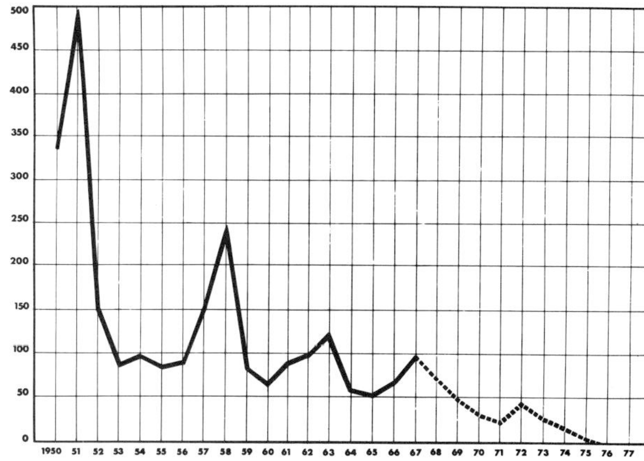

Above Graph showing the decline of smallpox throughout the world since 1950.

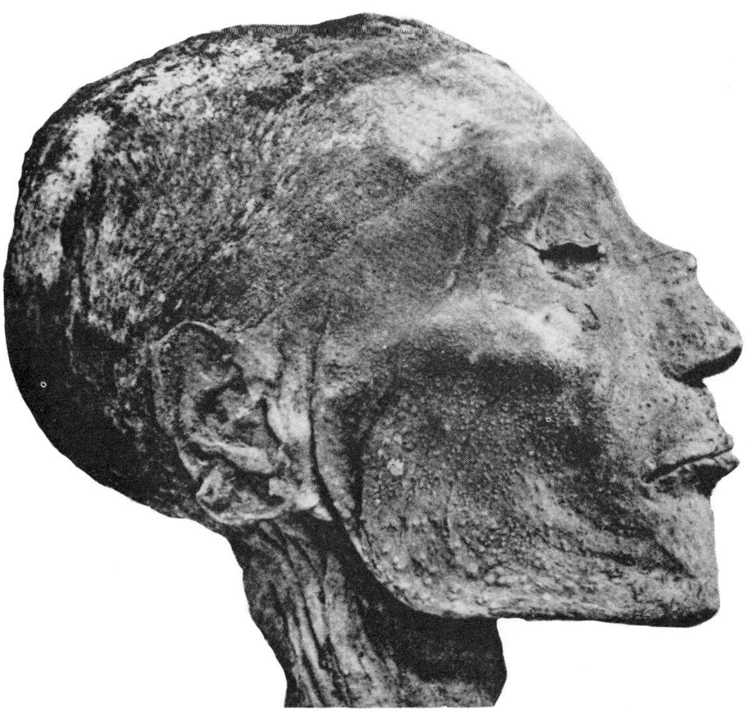

Left The mummified head of the Egyptian pharaoh Ramses V who died in 1160 B.C. Because of the small round bumps on the jaw, experts think he had smallpox.

1 *Jenner's Life*

Edward Jenner was born on 17th May 1749, and died on 26th January 1823. For most of his life he lived near the River Severn in the village of Berkeley, Gloucestershire, which was the scene of his practice as a country surgeon and of his work as a naturalist.

Only one description of Jenner's appearance has been handed down. It was written as a kind of literary snapshot by one of Jenner's friends, Edward Gardner. "His height was rather under the middle size, his person was robust, but active and well-formed. In his dress he was peculiarly neat . . . I had heard so much of him that I had no small curiosity to see him. He was dressed in a blue coat and yellow buttons, buckskins, well-polished jockey boots, with handsome silver spurs, and he carried a smart whip with a silver handle. His hair, after the fashion of the times, was done up in a club, and he wore a broad-brimmed hat."

Painting of scenes from Jenner's life. At the top is Berkeley vicarage where Jenner was born.

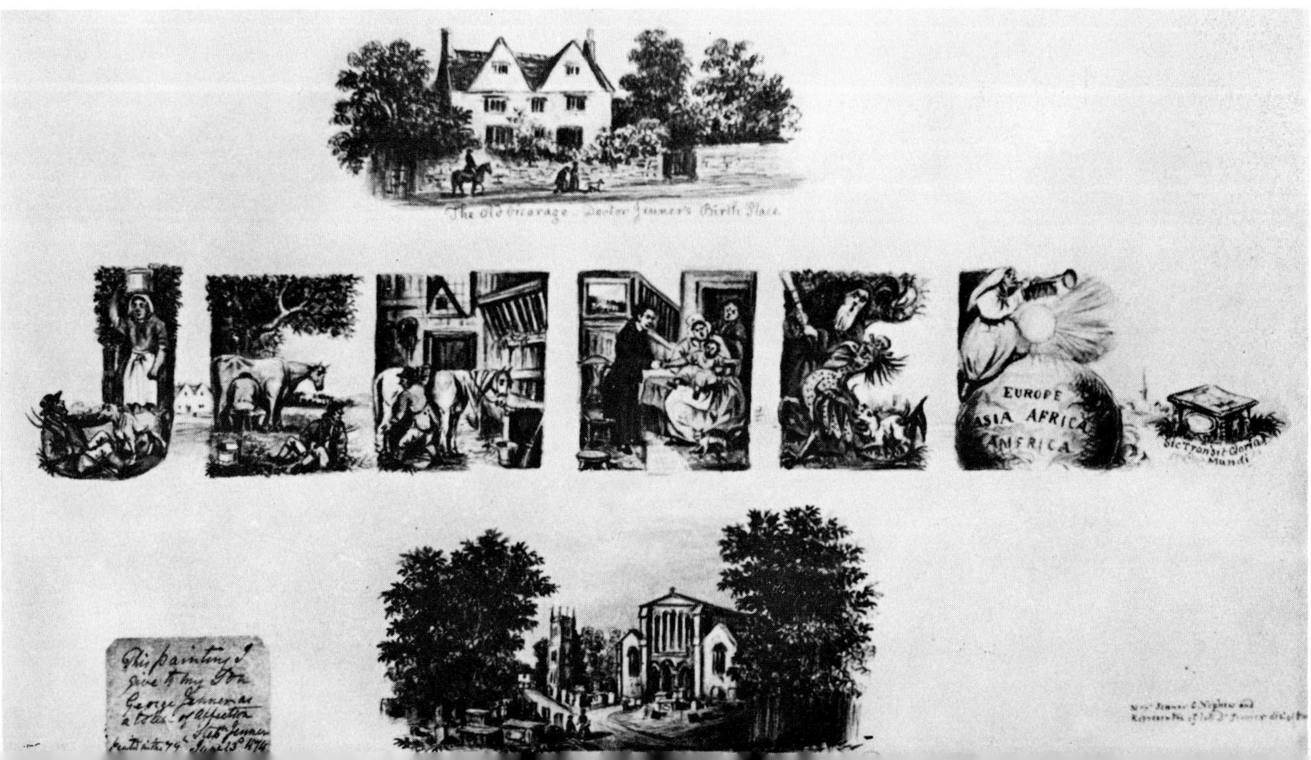

The Reverend and Mrs Stephen Jenner had ten children. Edward was the youngest. Edward's father was vicar of Berkeley and rector of the nearby village of Rockhampton close by the River Severn. The family had strong connections with the church and with farming. Edward's grandfather was the son of Squire Jenner of Slimbridge, now a centre for the Wildfowl Trust, while Mrs Jenner was the daughter of the previous vicar of Berkeley, the Reverend Henry Head. Edward's brothers Stephen and Henry read Divinity at Oxford. Stephen was to play a great part in shaping the future founder of vaccination, for after both his mother and his father died when Edward was five years old, Stephen came to the rescue and brought up his young brother. When Stephen became rector of the neighbouring village of Rockhampton, Edward went to live with him, while his sister remained at Berkeley where her husband was now vicar.

At the age of eight, Edward began school and when he was eleven went to Cirencester Grammar School. Here he was given an orthodox classical education—"and obtained a tolerable proficiency

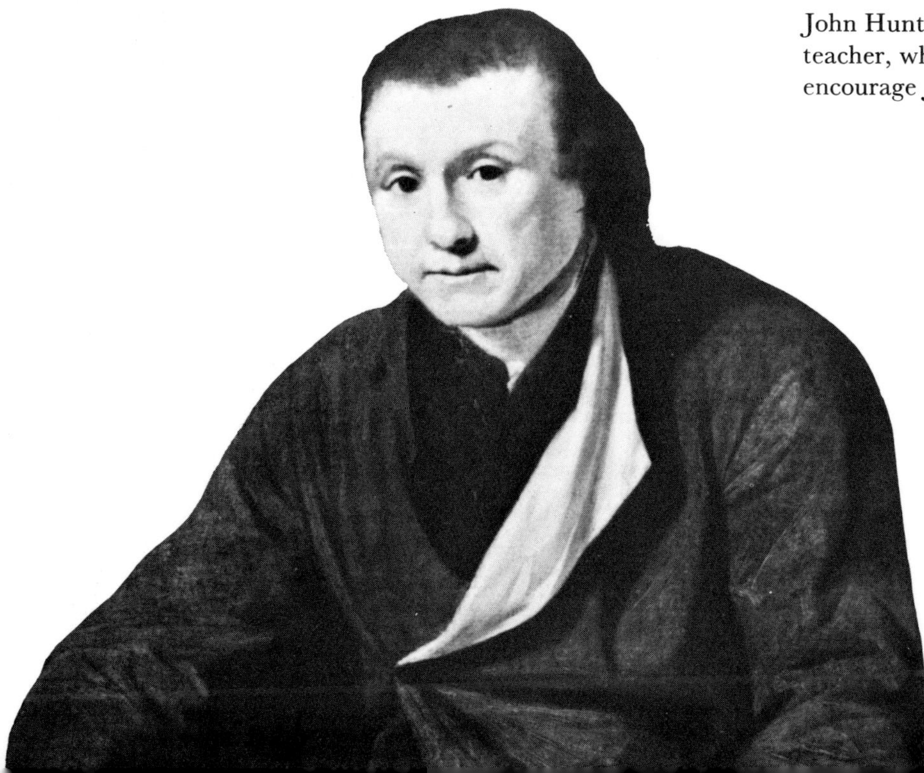

John Hunter, the great surgeon and teacher, who did so much to encourage Jenner's talents.

in the Latin language and got a decent smattering of Greek." Here he kept a collection of dormice and fossils.

It was probably Stephen who encouraged Edward to begin training as a country surgeon. He therefore began by being apprenticed at the age of twelve to Mr Ludlow, a country surgeon of Chipping Sodbury. He assisted Mr Ludlow in surgical operations and pharmacy and in helping with the running of the country practice. This was the form of medical training then in use.

To Stephen Jenner and to Mr Ludlow must go the credit for the decision to send Edward, at the age of twenty-one, to London to complete his medical studies under the guidance of the great surgeon-scientist and teacher, John Hunter. By this means Jenner gained the certificates of attendance at courses necessary to mark him as a bonafide surgeon so that he could set up his own practice. (It was not until 1858 that the General Medical Council was set up and the registration of legally qualified practitioners was begun.) During the two years of instruction a remarkable friendship and scientific communion between Jenner and Hunter developed, and which was to lead to Jenner's epoch-making discovery of the habits of the cuckoo, for which he was elected F.R.S.

Jenner returned to the Berkeley district in 1773 and began his work as a country practitioner of surgery and medicine. He was popular, and his friends enjoyed his conversation and travelling with him on his rounds to his patients in the surrounding villages and farms. He became an important member of two medical clubs which used to convene their meetings at hostelries in the area. It was at these meetings that Jenner pestered his friends with his early thoughts about using cow pox as a protection against smallpox. Poems, songs and music were also part of this period. His poetry and ballad-singing had some merit, and

A contemporary silhouette of Catherine, Jenner's wife.

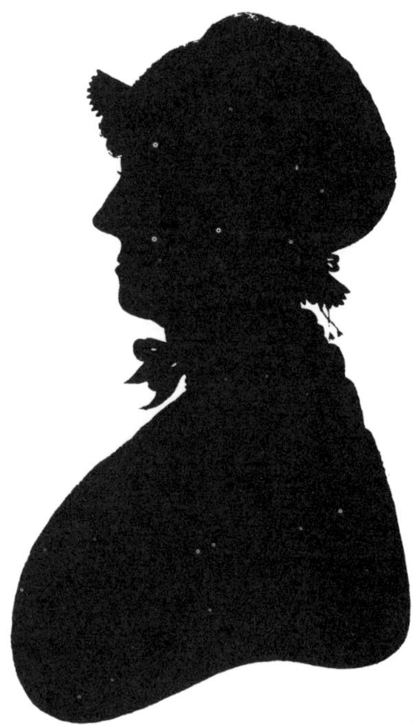

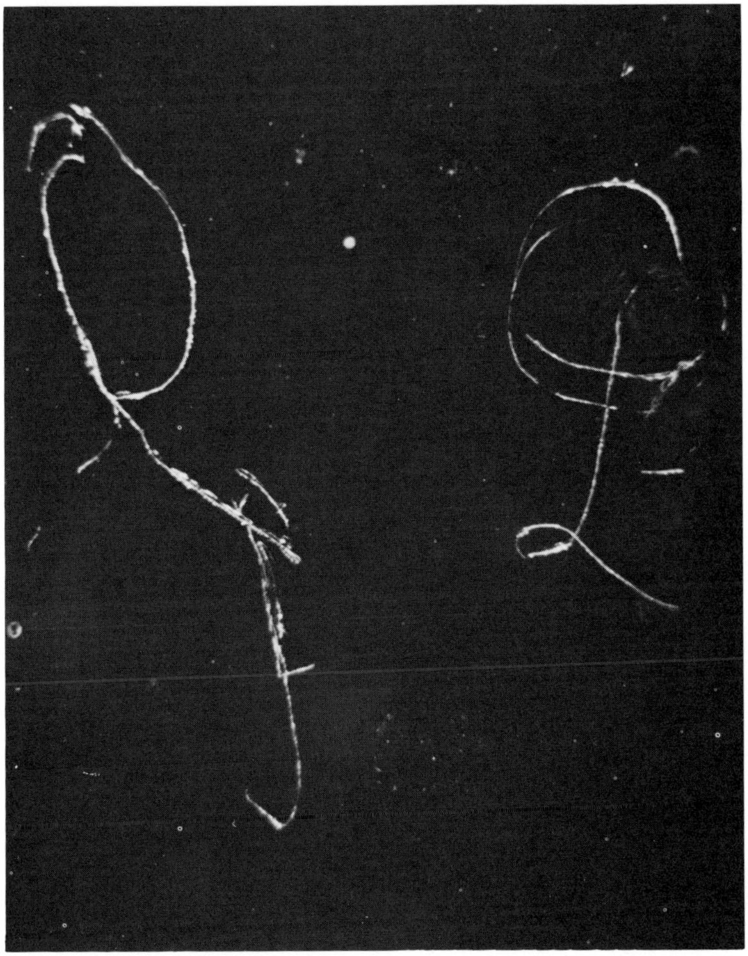

Initials scratched by Jenner's children on a window at the Chantry, their home at Berkeley, Gloucestershire.

he could play the flute and violin. Much of his work as a naturalist was done at this time.

Jenner seems to have had an unhappy love affair. The following letter, so often quoted, exactly expresses Hunter's human understanding of the situation, together with his glowing and fierce scientific passion: "Dear Jenner, I own that I was at a loss to account for your silence, and I was sorry at the cause. I can easily conceive how you must feel, for you have two passions to cope with; viz. that of being disappointed in love; and that of being defeated; both will wear out, perhaps the first soonest, and I want you to get a hedgehog, in the beginning of winter, and weigh him; put him in your garden, and let him have leaves, hay and straw to cover himself with, which he will do; then weigh him in the spring and see what he has lost. Ever yours, John Hunter. 25th September 1779."

In 1788, on 6th March, Edward Jenner married Catherine Kingscote from a village some ten miles away. The marriage was happy, and Catherine soon became active in establishing and running Sunday Schools. Edward and Catherine had two sons and a daughter. Unfortunately, the older son, Edward, was never very strong. He developed tuberculosis, and died in 1810 at the age of twenty-one. His brother Robert was more fortunate, and after going to Exeter College, Oxford, went into the Army and rose to the rank of Colonel. Jenner's daughter, Catherine, stayed to look after her father after his wife's death in 1815. Catherine married a solicitor, and went to live in Edgbaston, Birmingham.

When John Hunter died in 1793, it was not Jenner's only loss on the scientific side of his life, for his nephew George, who had been his assistant, left to work in Newfoundland with a medical missionary friend, the Reverend John Clinch. In 1795, Jenner and his family were involved in an epidemic of typhus (or typhoid) fever. Jenner only just survived, but his brother Henry died. His nephew Stephen was lost at sea when a troopship on the way to the Peninsular War, foundered on Chesil Beach, Dorset (a notorious area for wrecking and looting).

But in spite of these family disasters Jenner was able to promote his enquiry into the definition of the disease of cows called cow pox, and its use by inoculation into the human as a means of preventing smallpox. The first successful preventive inoculation, later called vaccination, was performed by Jenner on 14th May 1796.

For the rest of his life, in addition to running his practice, he was concerned with the national and international adoption of correct cow pox vaccination. Jenner survived his wife by seven years and continued preaching precise vaccination methods, and in the field of natural history he returned to his earlier work on the migration of birds, and made some original observations. By now Extraordinary Physician to the King, he was made Mayor of Berkeley and Justice of the Peace. In the summer of 1820 he had a stroke, from which he recovered without disability or paralysis.

On a freezing morning on 24th January 1823, Jenner walked to a neighbouring village to arrange for the distribution of fuel to the poor. He seemed to be all right. The next morning he was found on the floor of his library, unconscious from another stroke. His right side was paralyzed, and he died on 26th January.

He is buried beside his wife in Berkeley Church.

2 *Jenner's World*

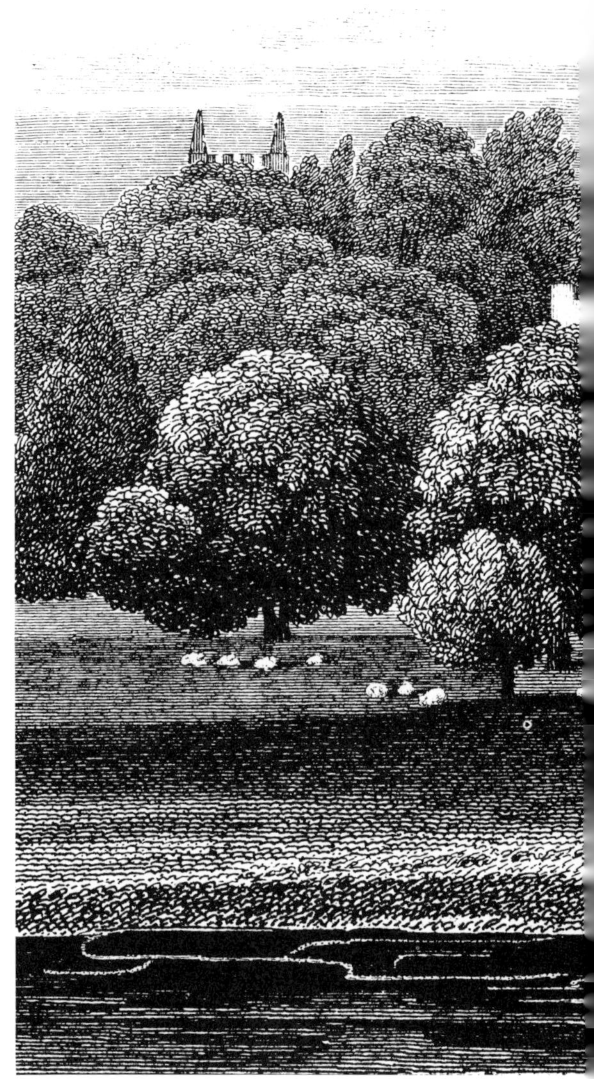

Berkeley Castle, home of the earls of Berkeley and scene of the murder of Edward II.

Berkeley is known chiefly for three things. It is the place where King Edward II was murdered in Berkeley Castle in 1327; the place where Edward Jenner first started to vaccinate people, and where today there is an atomic power station. Berkeley features so much in the amazing discoveries of Jenner and in shaping his attitude towards life and the role he chose to play, that it is helpful to give a brief account of it.

Berkeley lies in the centre of low lying rich pastureland near the eastern bank of the River Severn, between the river and the road connecting Gloucester and Bristol. Cheltenham is to the north and Bath is to the south. Five miles or so to the east lies the high escarpment of the Cotswold Hills.

Geologically, the area is of special interest, and Jenner became a local expert on its formations and fossils. On the banks of the Severn he would pick up specimens of the large curled fossils of pre-historic ammonites, or the smaller molluscs known as "devil's toe-nails."

Jenner was born into the country scene at Berkeley, with its constant change of seasons, its rich pasturelands, its orchards, wildlife and fossils. He describes the basic pastoral life of the period in his poem *Berkeley Fair*—about a fair granted in perpetuity in 1394 to be held on Hollirood day in May.

"The sun drove off the twilight gray,
And promised all a cloudless day;
His yellow beams glanced o'er the dews,
And changed to gems their pearly hues,
The song birds on every spray,
And sang as if they knew the day;
The blackbird piped his mellow note;

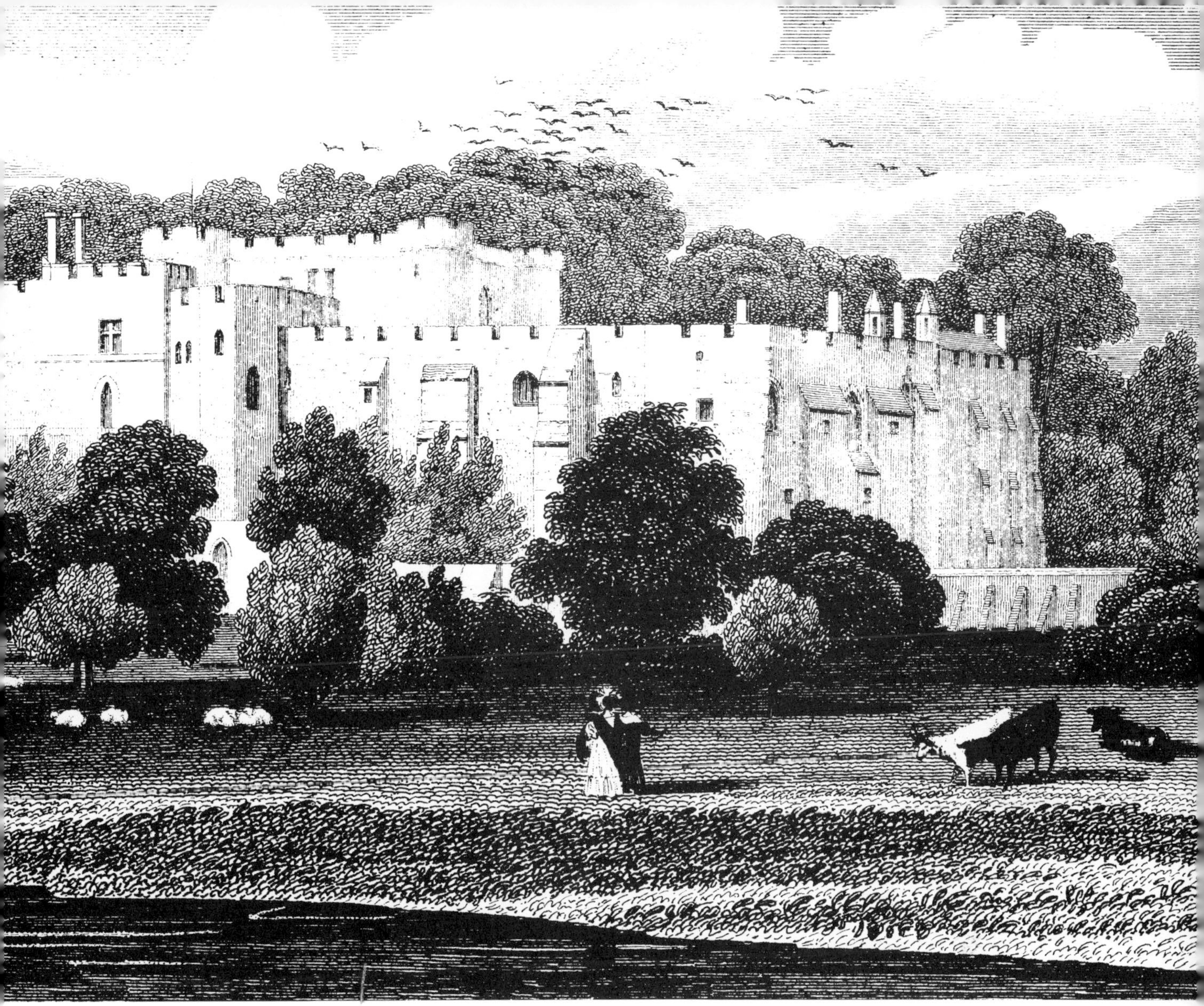

The goldfinch strained his downy throat;
The little wren, too, left her nest,
And striving, sang her very best;
The robin wisely kept away,
His song too plaintive for the day
'Twas *Berkeley Fair,* and nature's smile
Spread joy around for many a mile."

Berkeley has been subject to extremes of weather

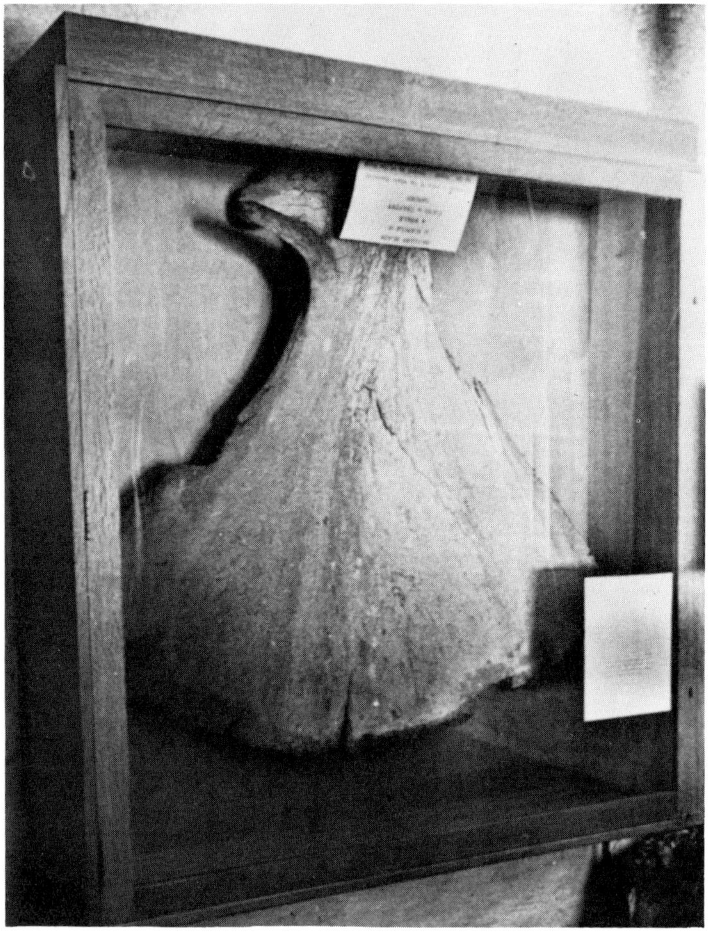

Bone from a whale washed up at Berkeley and dissected by Jenner.

and tides. There were flood disasters in 1606 and 1703. In 1620 a large whale was washed up on the tide. A smaller whale was washed up in Jenner's day and he cut it up and sent it in a coach to John Hunter in London.

The winters could be very cold. The following account of Jenner's ride to Kingscote is probably the earliest record of the effects of hypothermia and exposure, effects much in the public eye today when parties of school children are trapped and lost on hills and moorlands in snow conditions. The account also contains what must be the earliest reference to the precautions to be taken in the first aid treatment of frostbite; rapid rewarming causes gangrene through cell death and coagulation, therefore slow warming is essential.

Blizzard on the Cotswolds—3rd January 1786.

"The air felt more intensely cold than I ever remember to have experienced it. The ground was deeply covered with snow, and it blew quite a hurricane, accompanied with continual snow. Being well clothed, I did not find the cold made much impression on me till I ascended the hills . . . There was no possibility of keeping the snow from drifting under my hat, so that half of my face and my neck was, for a long time, wrapt in ice . . . I had still two miles to go. As the sense of external cold increased, the heat about the stomach seemed to increase. I had the same sensations as if I had drunk a considerable quantity of wine or brandy; and my spirits rose in proportion to this sensation.

"I felt . . . like one intoxicated . . . My hands at last grew extremely painful, and this distressed my spirits in some degree. When I came to the house I was unable to dismount without assistance. I was almost senseless; but I had just recollection and power enough left to prevent the servants from bringing me to a fire . . . I could bear no greater heat than that of the stable for some time. Rubbing my hands in snow took off the pain quickly. The parts which had been most benumbed, felt for some time as if they had been slightly burnt. My horse lost part of the cuticle and hair at the upper part of the neck, and also from his ears. I had not the least inclination to take wine, or any kind of refreshment."

In 1788 Jenner acquired Chantry House, and this became his main home for the rest of his life. Modestly he called the Chantry a cottage, but even by present day standards it is a fine house of fifteen rooms in a lovely setting. Among the trees near the churchyard Jenner's Temple of Vaccinia is to be found, a rustic

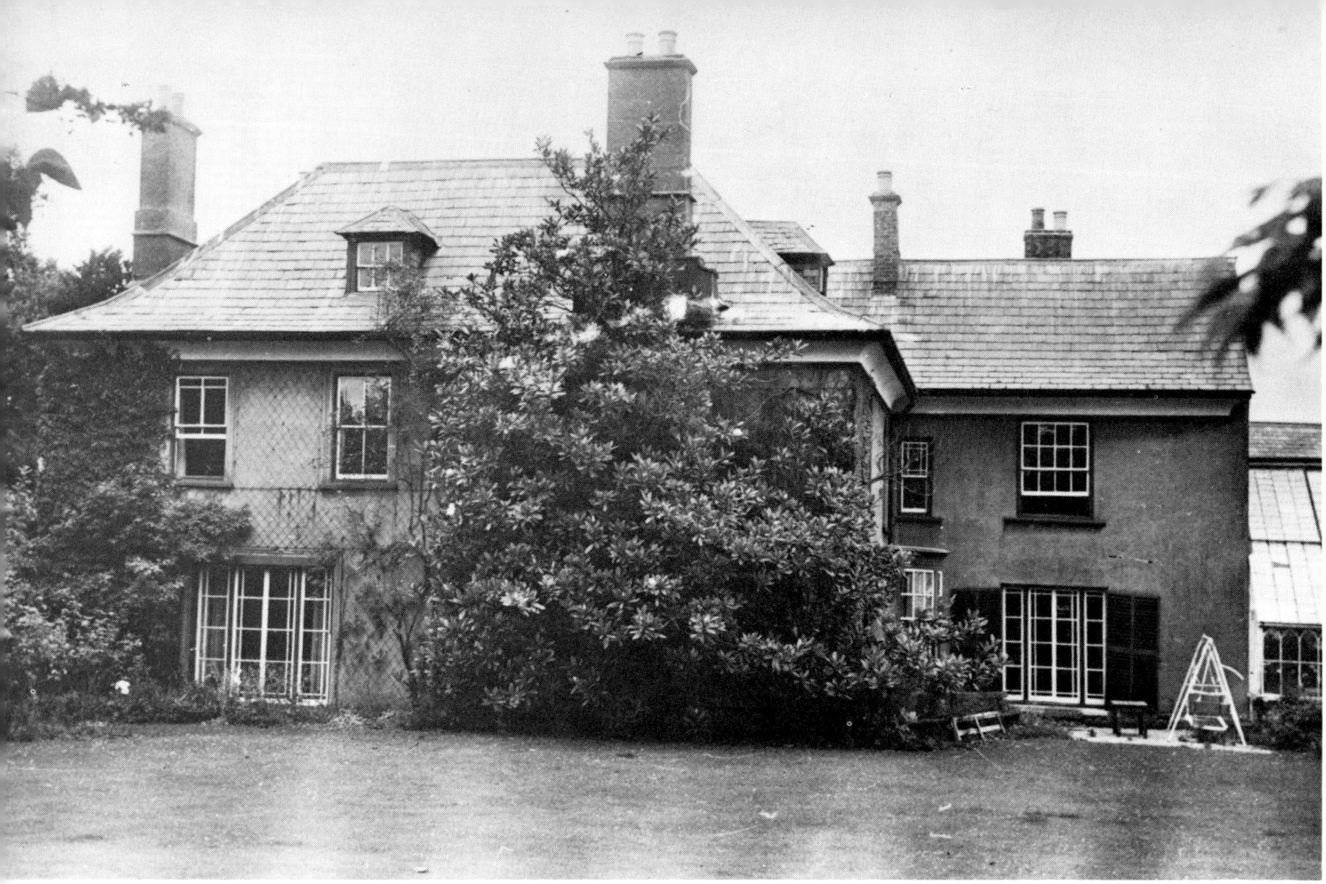

and thatched one-room building, where he used to vaccinate all comers. Close by is the house Jenner built for James Phipps on whom he carried out the first historic vaccination. This house now contains a small museum.

Jenner was always afforded support and encouragement by the Berkeley family. This family had also been associated with another great discovery of medical science, that of the circulation of the blood by William Harvey in 1628. The Earl of Berkeley was Harvey's patron.

It has been said that Jenner and his work would have received even greater publicity and rewards if he had been born either earlier or later. Had this been so he would have missed the vital training and guidance of John Hunter, and the loss of life from smallpox added to the wars and revolutions of those

Above The Chantry, Berkeley, the home of Jenner and his family. *Opposite* The Temple of Vaccinia, the small rustic summerhouse at Berkeley where Jenner carried out vaccinations.

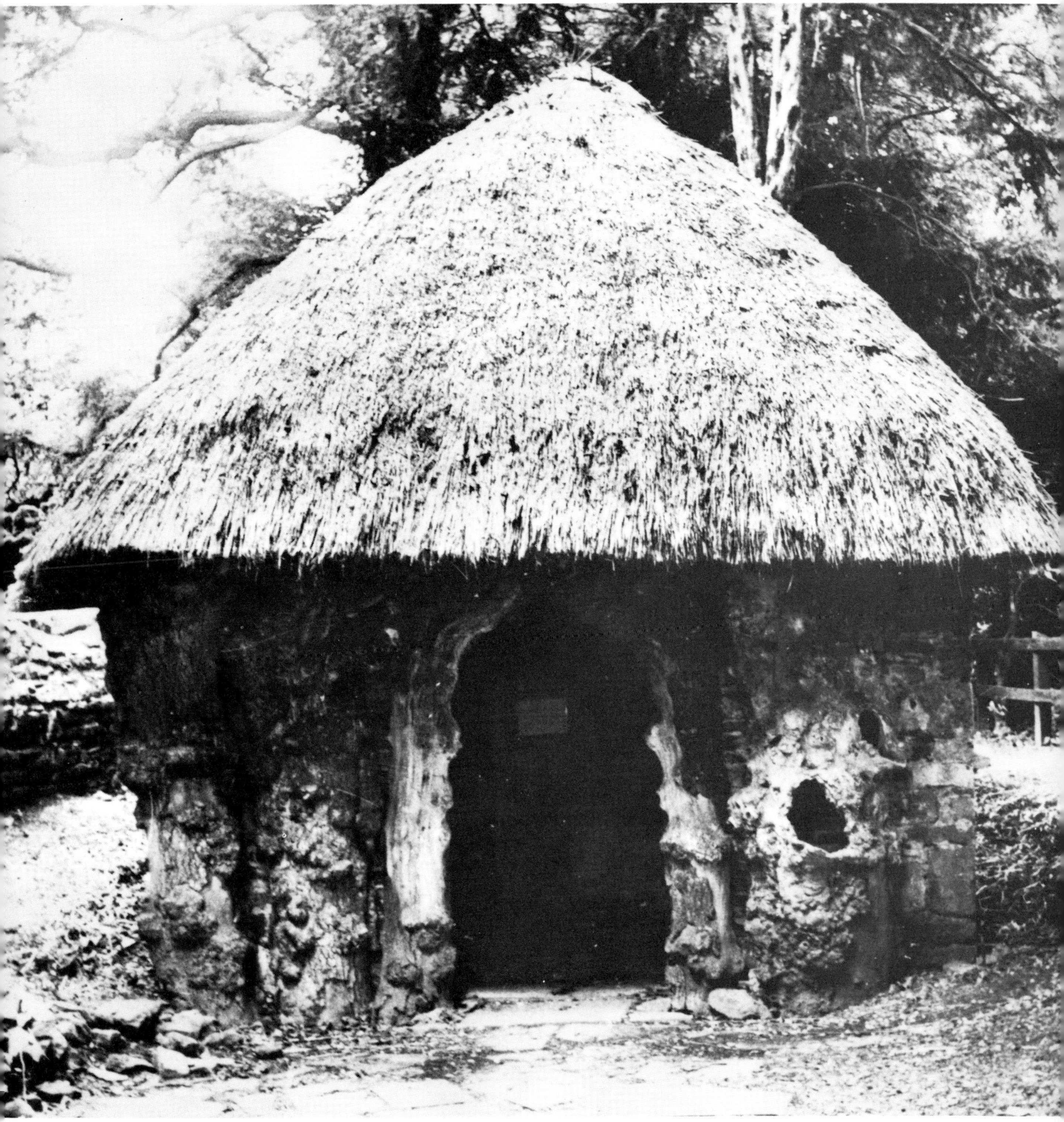

days would have been all the greater.

When Jenner was a child, William Pitt the Elder united English and Scots to fight a dramatic four years' war which culminated in the founding of the first British Empire. Jenner was a schoolboy when Robert Clive, aged 24, previously a clerk in the East India Company, first displayed his military genius. After the episode of the Black Hole of Calcutta in 1756, Clive became master of Bengal and the possessor of a fortune of £250,000. In contrast Jenner in his campaign for vaccination saved millions of lives and was lucky to receive £30,000 (less £1,000 tax).

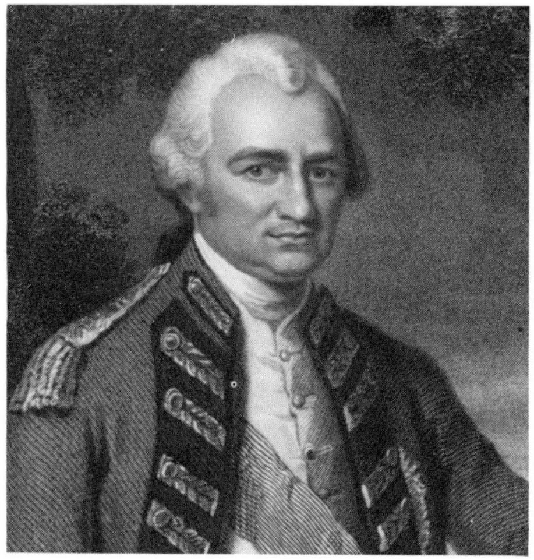

Above Robert Clive, who achieved fame and fortune in India when Jenner was a boy.

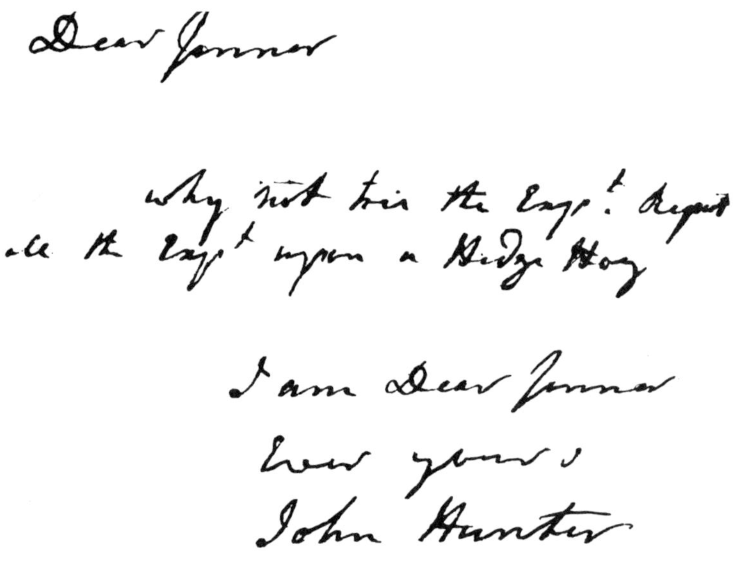

Dear Jenner

why not try the Expt. Repeat all the Expt upon a Hedge Hog

I am Dear Jenner
Ever yours
John Hunter

Left Letter from Hunter to Jenner about the experiments with hedgehogs.

The period of Jenner's tuition in London under John Hunter coincided with Captain Cook's return from Australia, the governorship of famine stricken Bengal by Warren Hastings, and the trouble brewing in the American colonies. While the American colonies were being lost, Jenner and Hunter were studying hedgehogs, hibernation, and the habits of the cuckoo. William Pitt the Younger became Prime Minister at the age of 24, and intro-

Opposite The title-page of *An Inquiry Into Cow Pox,* Jenner's most important work. The comparative rarity of smallpox in the world today is a tribute to its author's brilliance.

AN

INQUIRY

INTO

THE CAUSES AND EFFECTS

OF

THE VARIOLÆ VACCINÆ,

A DISEASE

DISCOVERED IN SOME OF THE WESTERN COUNTIES OF ENGLAND,

PARTICULARLY

GLOUCESTERSHIRE,

AND KNOWN BY THE NAME OF

THE COW POX.

BY EDWARD JENNER, M. D. F. R. S. &c.

——— QUID NOBIS CERTIUS IPSIS
SENSIBUS ESSE POTEST, QUO VERA AC FALSA NOTEMUS.

LUCRETIUS.

London:

PRINTED, FOR THE AUTHOR,

BY SAMPSON LOW, N°. 7, BERWICK STREET, SOHO:

AND SOLD BY LAW, AVE-MARIA LANE; AND MURRAY AND HIGHLEY, FLEET STREET.

1798.

duced the Budget and founded the science of business management. Jenner had only just been elected a Fellow of the Royal Society when the Bastille was stormed on 14th July 1789. His twenty years of country doctoring and natural history research therefore took place between the beginning of one revolution in America and another in France.

The first successful vaccination in 1796 was in the year of Napoleon's first victories in Italy. The *Inquiry into Cow Pox* was published in the year of the battle of the Nile. Jenner's wife died in 1815 and Jenner died two years after Napoleon.

During Jenner's remaining years, Sir Stamford Raffles founded Singapore and the London Zoo, and consulted Jenner about his experiences with John Hunter's famous menagerie at Earl's Court. In the year of Jenner's death the Monroe doctrine ("hands off America") was propounded.

Two more revolutions were to feature in Jenner's life—the Industrial Revolution and that in chemical science. While he was a student Jenner was to hear of the development of the mechanization of spinning cotton and wool associated with the names of Hargreaves, Arkwright, Crompton and Cartwright. In the Soho area of Birmingham, James Watt and Matthew Boulton developed their engineering business after Watt had invented his steam engine in 1769. Soho was also to nurture the invention of William Murdock—gaslight from coal. The first encouraging results of the vaccination campaign were beginning to come in when the first steamship, the *Charlotte Dundas*, moved on the waters of the Clyde in 1802. Further developments of these inventions, the Stockton and Darlington railway in 1825 and the first steamship crossing of the Atlantic in 1826, were to come just after Jenner's death.

Jenner, in a project with the Earl of Berkeley and Gardner, built a balloon in the Great Hall at Berkeley Castle, took it to the Castle meadow, and

Henry Cavendish, discoverer of the gas hydrogen.

filled it with hydrogen. It made a spectacular flight to Symonds Hall ten miles away. It was refilled at Kingscote Park for another successful flight. Thus Jenner became one of the first experimental balloonists.

Cavendish's discovery of hydrogen was followed by that of oxygen by Priestley and Scheele in 1774, and Sir Humphry Davy discovered nitrous oxide as well as inventing the miner's safety-lamp. A Dr Beddoes, a chemist, had set up a Medical Pneumatic Institute (1799) for the treatment of chest diseases by the inhalation of oxygen and Davy's nitrous oxide (laughing gas). The apparatus was designed by James Watt, and associates included Dr Erasmus Darwin—grandfather of Charles Darwin—the poets William Wordsworth, Samuel Coleridge and Robert Southey, a member of the Wedgewood family and Paul Roget (later secretary of the Royal Society and compiler of the *Thesaurus*).

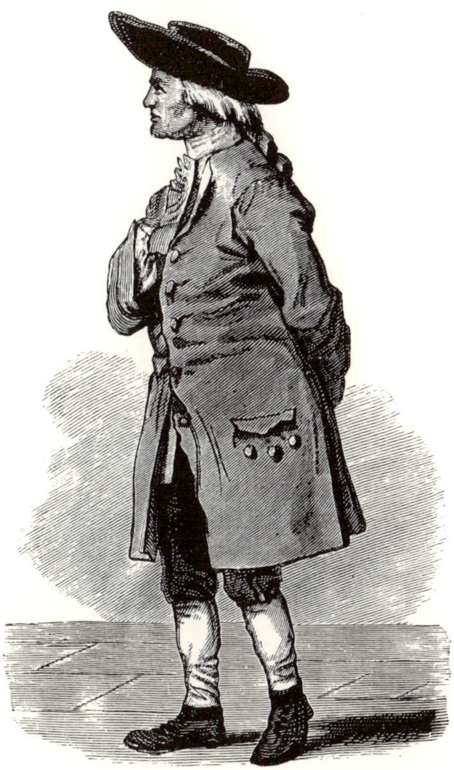

Possibly it was the gas adventure which brought Davy and Jenner together. They became firm friends and continued Jenner's work on the migration of birds. Davy helped to present his paper to the Royal Society after Jenner's death. Jenner and Davy form a link between John Hunter and Michael Faraday. As Hunter was Jenner's guiding genius, so Humphry Davy gave Michael Faraday a chance as a lab boy and then fostered his development as the founder of the revolution in electro-magnetism.

Also in the context of the chemical revolution it would not be amiss to mention Jenner's early and lasting interest in chemistry. He devised a method of purifying tartar emetic by recrystallization so that accurate dosage and a predictable effect could be achieved. This was one of the earliest ventures into the quality control of a product. In later years Jenner returned again to the effects of this chemical and particularly its use in treating skin diseases. Curiously, an ointment containing tartar emetic can

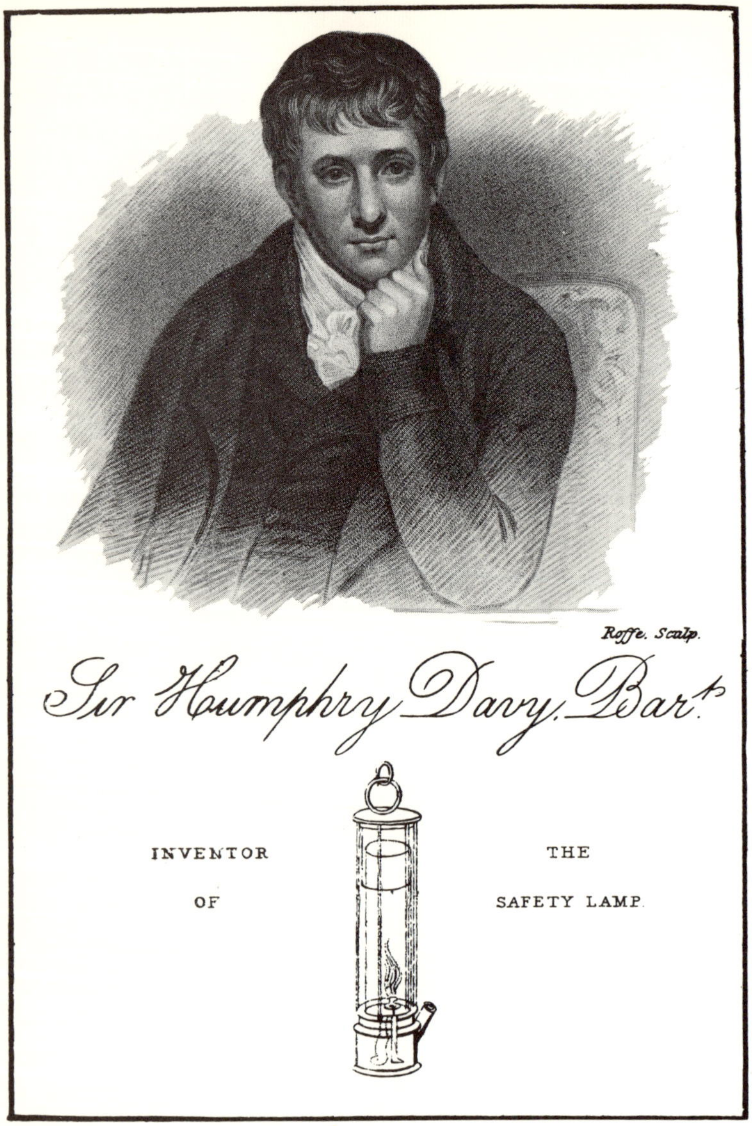
Roffe. Sculp.
Sir Humphry Davy, Bart.
INVENTOR
OF
THE
SAFETY LAMP.

Humphry Davy who discovered nitrous oxide (laughing gas). He also invented the miner's safety lamp which did much to help the miners in the appalling conditions of nineteenth century mines.

produce a skin eruption similar to smallpox!

It is interesting that Jenner and Pasteur, who was one year old when Jenner died, both began their scientific adventures through a study of crystals. While it was his researches on fermentation and vaccines that led to the foundation of the sciences of bacteriology and immunology, Pasteur's debut was as discoverer of the isomerism of tartaric acid crystals separating the dextro-rotatory from the laevo-rotatory forms.

Just as a review of scientific discovery in Jenner's day helps to place Jenner's contributions in relation to the work of others, a consideration of the literary scene is also helpful in understanding something of Jenner's personality, especially as he was such an active writer himself.

Jenner's life extended approximately from the deaths of Swift and Bach to the births of Tolstoy, Jules Verne and Walt Whitman.

Among Jenner's exact, or almost exact, contemporaries we can number Blake, Boswell, Burns, Byron, Goethe, and Sheridan. His older contemporaries include Gibbon, Goldsmith, Johnson, Kant and Sterne. Younger contemporaries, many of whom may well have owed their lives to Jenner's introduction of vaccination, include Jane Austen, Balzac, the Brontës, Carlyle, Coleridge, Fennimore Cooper, Dickens, Dostoevsky, Leigh Hunt, Ruskin, Tennyson and Wordsworth.

As far as we know the only major poet who came in contact with Jenner was Coleridge who wrote to ask if he could compose a laudatory poem about his hero. We are told that Jenner demurred. Jenner himself was an amateur poet. The extract from his poem *Berkeley Fair* illustrates his flair and his description of the pastoral life at Berkeley. Another poem is perhaps the only detailed poem which accurately describes weather forecasting. About fifty Jennerian poems are known. There is a unique collection of these in the University of Virginia.

Jenner also composed an essay in psychology, "Classes of the Human Powers of Intellect." It is hard to understand how a country surgeon and practitioner, with all his visiting to be done on horseback, found time to compose poetry, to make scientific observations on differing aspects of natural history, to arrange the publication of scientific pamphlets, and to write hundreds of letters.

3 *Jenner and Hunter*

Any account of Jenner's background as a surgeon and naturalist and the introduction of vaccination is incomplete without reference to John Hunter, the great surgeon and teacher, who trained him to care for his patients and also to think and experiment.

John Hunter was born in 1728. He came to London in 1748 and assisted his brother William at the Windmill anatomy school. John dissected the bodies of felons and also bodies removed from graves after burial by "body-snatchers" or "resurrectionists." He displayed such a gift for anatomy that William made him a partner in 1753. Later, John refused to go to Oxford as a medical student. "They wanted to make an old woman of me and stuff me with Latin and learning . . ."

From his experience as an army surgeon in dealing with the wounded in an expedition to Belle Isle, Hunter began his first of many treatises, that on gunshot wounds. He later set himself up in practice as a surgeon and in order to live and follow his developing interest in natural history and pathology (study of diseases) he began to take pupils.

In 1764 he rented a home at Earls Court on the site of the present railway station which was then in the open country. Here he assembled his rapidly expanding collection of specimens including the skeleton of the giant O'Brien, and here he ran a menagerie of all kinds of wild animals (a fore-runner of the London Zoo). He married Anne Home in 1771. Then, by buying two houses back to back in Leicester Square and Castle Street, he fitted out a residence for pupils, a lecture theatre, museum and workrooms—almost, one might say, he had his own medical school. He worked at a tremendous pace and never spared himself. He was always hard up, because all

William Hunter, brother of John and founder of the well-known Windmill anatomy school.

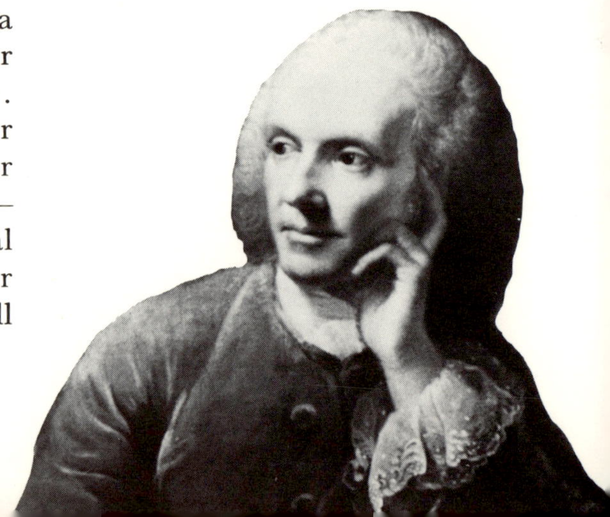

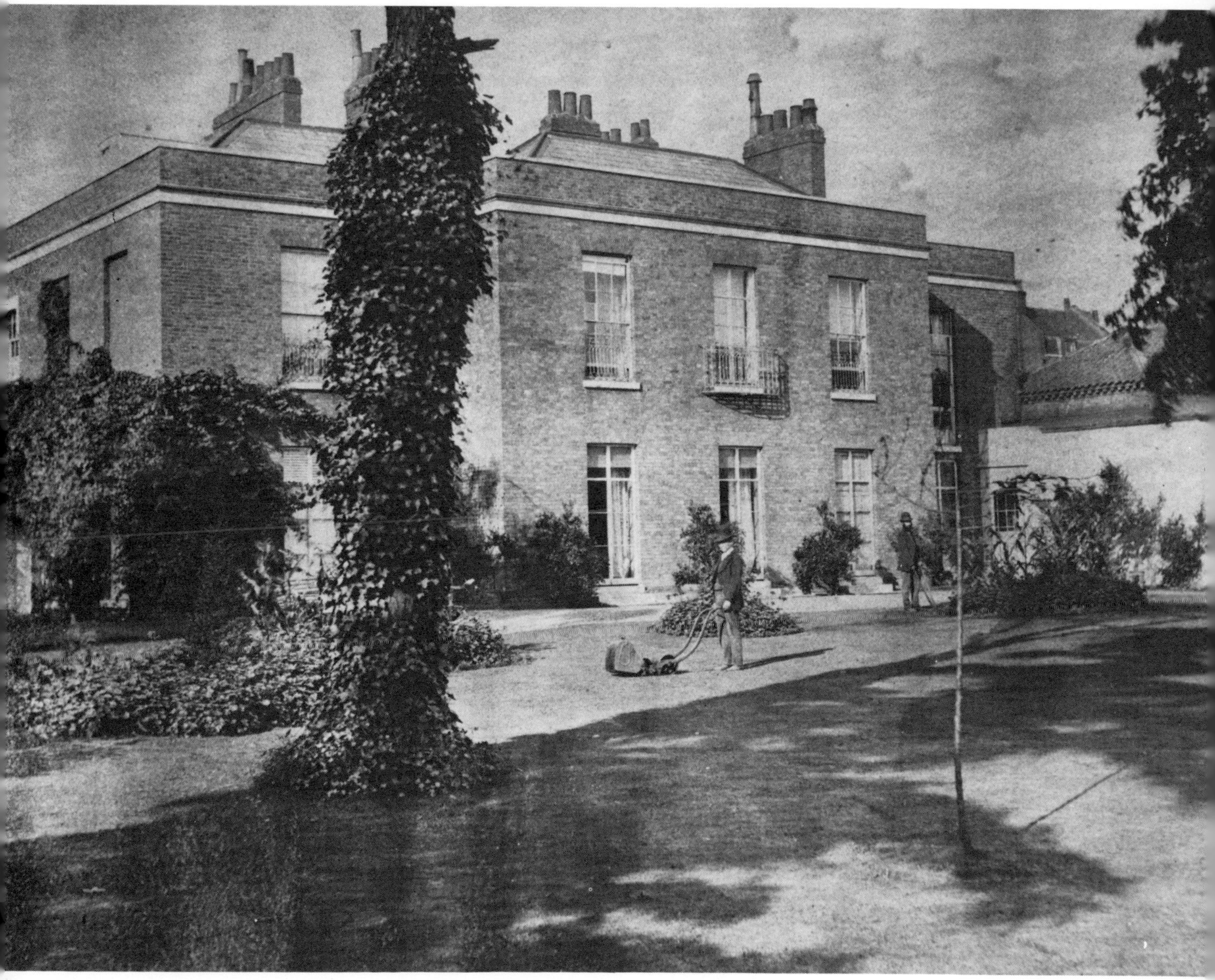

Earl's Court House, the home of John Hunter. When he moved there in 1764 it was in the country some way out of London, now it is the site of a London tube station.

his funds went on his research and, so it is said, on making his great collection (Jenner was one of his greatest suppliers). Today the remains of his collection is housed in a museum in the Royal College of Surgeons, where visitors come to view the skeleton of the Irish giant or Hunter's original experiments on transplantation. In 1777 Hunter developed angina pectoris and died suddenly in 1793. It has been estimated that he taught anatomy and pathology to about 1,000 pupils, including many who became leaders of surgery at home and abroad.

Edward Jenner was invited to become Hunter's first house pupil. The hours of work were long and hard—assisting Hunter in his work at St. George's Hospital and in the practice, attending anatomy, pathology, pharmacy and midwifery lectures and helping Hunter with his research in the evenings. It was in these intense two years that a remarkable comradeship and understanding developed between these two men. For the rest of his life Jenner would refer to Hunter as "the dear man." Baron, Jenner's official biographer, says "The pupil not only respected the teacher, but he loved the man; there was in both, a directness and plainness of conduct, an unquenchable desire for knowledge, and a congenial love of truth."

By December 1772 Jenner had collected all his certificates for attendance "with diligence" at courses on anatomy, surgery, materia medica (pharmacy) chemistry and midwifery. Later Jenner acquired the M.D. from Aberdeen, and, after vaccination was a success, honorary degrees of M.D. from Oxford, LL.D. from Harvard, and other diplomas. There was talk of election to membership or fellowship of the College of Physicians in London but Jenner was requested at the age of sixty to take a preliminary examination in Latin. He said: "I would not do it for a diadem. That indeed would be a bauble. I would not do it for John Hunter's museum and that, you will allow, is no trifle."

Jenner's diligence was plainly obvious soon after he started work under Hunter. Captain Cook had just returned from his circumnavigation of the world. Joseph Banks, who later became President of the Royal Society, had collected many natural history specimens. Jenner was asked to catalogue and classify these. He did this so well that he was invited to accompany Cook's next expedition as naturalist, but he declined.

Jenner's ability was such that he received a personal request by John Hunter to become his partner in surgery, research and teaching in London; but Jenner still wished to return to the Berkeley countryside. Also, a merchant offered Jenner a post in the East Indies after being very impressed by the young surgeon at a dinner party in Bath, during which there was discussion as to which part of a candle flame was the hottest. Applying Hunters dictum—"Why think, why not try the experiment?" —Jenner inserted his finger into the base of the flame and was able to retain it there for a short while, but on placing his finger just above the flame he had to withdraw it immediately saying, "There gentlemen, the question is settled."

There is a sad ending to this story of Jenner's diligence under Hunter. Jenner was the first to describe the degenerative changes which occur in the coronary arteries of the heart.

He had detected these when performing post-mortem examinations on patients who died after suffering from a pain in the chest after exercise—named angina pectoris by Heberden. In 1777 Jenner learned that Hunter was beginning to suffer from angina pectoris. Jenner in writing to Heberden about his discovery of the diseased coronary arteries says: "How much the heart must suffer from [the coronary arteries] not being able to perform their functions [we cannot be surprised at the painful spasms] is a subject I need not enlarge upon; therefore I shall only remark that it is possible that all the symptoms may arise from this one circumstance."

Jenner could not tell Hunter what he believed to be wrong with him: "I am fearful if Mr H. should admit this, that it may deprive him of his hopes of recovery." In fact, Hunter died after an argument with his colleagues concerning students' privileges on 16th October 1793.

John Hunter, so important to Jenner, was as near perfect as a surgeon could be because he:—

(1) cared for his patients,
(2) studied and kept up to date so that his patients would benefit,
(3) carried out basic scientific research for the greater understanding of the meaning of structure, function and disease which would, in the long run, benefit humanity, and
(4) handed on the torch.

Over a century later the American medical educationist, Simon Flexner, was to preach these four essentials, but Hunter was the embodiment of them all—and it was he who handed the torch on to a thousand young men, including Edward Jenner.

4 *The Natural Historian*

The years between the return of Edward Jenner to Berkeley in 1773 and the death of John Hunter in 1793 were years of a growing practice as a country surgeon and of natural history research.

At first Jenner continued to help John Hunter in his research and in building up the fantastic Hunterian collection of natural history. Hunter wanted to find out everything about the hibernation of animals. He had obtained a new measuring device, a thermometer, and considered that the measurement of body-core temperatures was essential to understanding survival. He looked to Jenner as his supplier of live specimens and collaborator. In his paper to the Royal Society he says: "As I was unable to procure hedgehogs in the torpid state . . . I got my friend Mr Jenner, surgeon, at Berkeley to make the same experiments in that animal that I might compare them with those in the dormouse, and his account is as follows . . ."

One of Jenner's experiments was to find that at 30°F the animal had no desire for food, but on warming to 93°F it seized a toad, and immediately ate some bread and milk.

Hunter also got Jenner to measure core temperatures of vegetables standing in the fields during winter.

This period of the joint work on hibernation was marked on 2nd August 1775 by Hunter's immortal letter to Jenner (and to posterity): "I thank you for your experiment with the hedgehog; but why do you ask me a question by way of solving it? I think your solution is just; *but why think, why not try the experiment?* Repeat all the experiments upon a hedgehog as soon as you can, and they will give you the solution."

Jenner helped Hunter in other investigations. He had told Hunter about the occasional appearance of calves who were bisexual (with ovary and testis), called freemartins, and Hunter later read a paper to the Royal Society on this phenomenon. Another paper to the Royal Society was about the relationship of the wolf and the jackal to the dog—the same species, Jenner had reported: "The little jackal-bitch which you gave me is grown a fine handsome animal; but she certainly does not possess the understanding of common dogs. She is easily lost when I take her out, and is quite inattentive to a whistle. She is more shy than a dog, and starts frequently when a quick motion is made before her. Of her inches she is uncommonly fleet, much more so than any dog I ever saw."

When a small whale was washed up with her progeny on the banks of the River Severn, Hunter wrote to say how the specimens were to be prepared for transport to London in a coach. Jenner and Mr Ludlow found the whale's milk rich like cows' milk with added cream. Hunter also asked them to find out if it went sour.

Other letters from Hunter included various demands and ideas:

"If you catch any bats, let me have some of them."

"I received your salmon and very fresh . . ."

"I will also take any fossils you may send me . . ."

"What do you think of examining eels? Their sexes have not been found out . . ."

Soon after Jenner's return to Berkeley Hunter encouraged Jenner to study the cuckoo. Eventually Jenner sent Hunter his draft manuscript on the habits of the cuckoo in the form of a letter, which contained several original observations. Cuckoos begin to arrive about 17th April, and it is the male cuckoo which has the distinctive call. Cuckoos do not pair: the female is promiscuous. She produces a

Jenner's observations led to the discovery that female cuckoos make no nests, but lay their eggs in the nests of other small birds who then have to hatch out the baby cuckoos.

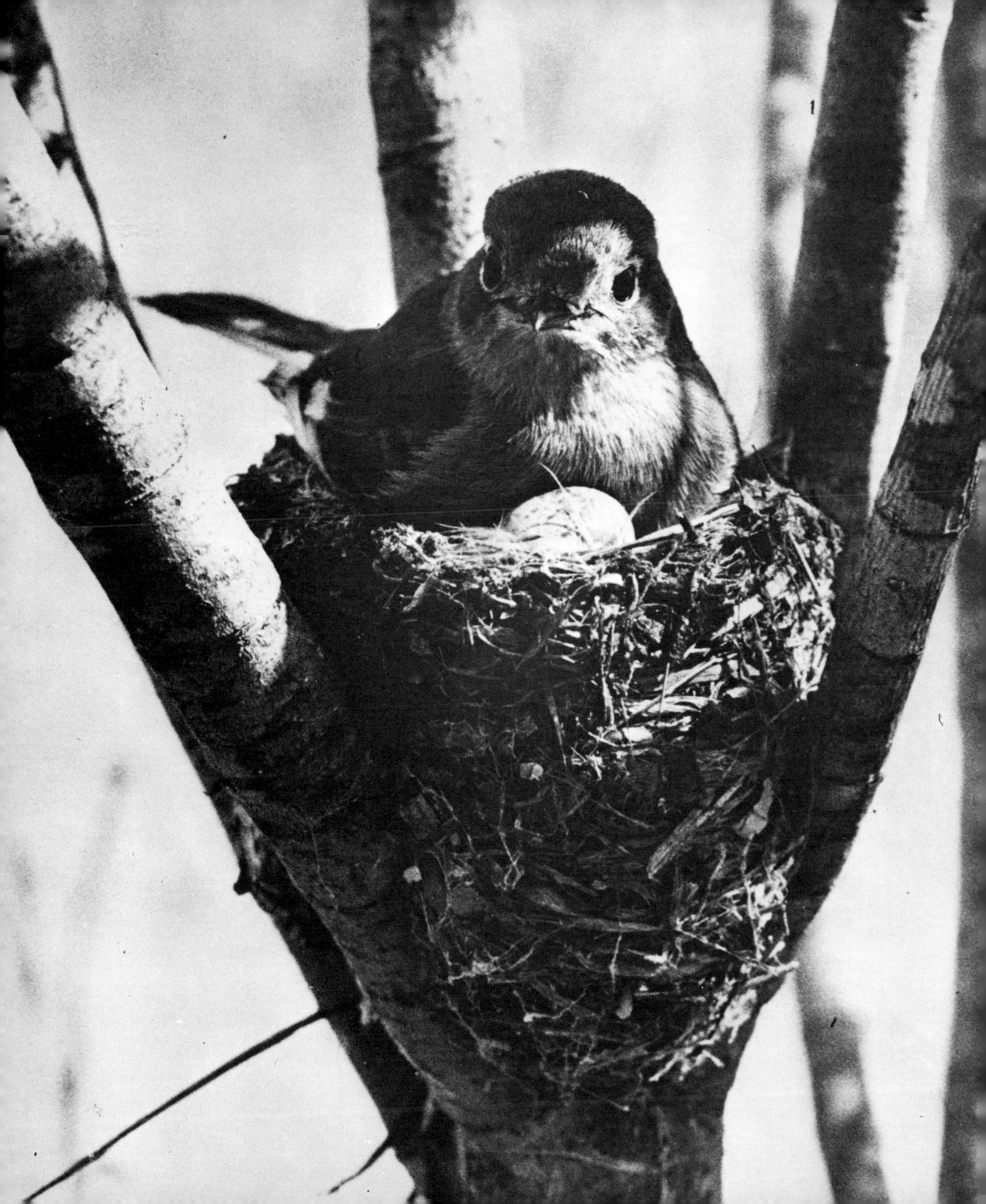

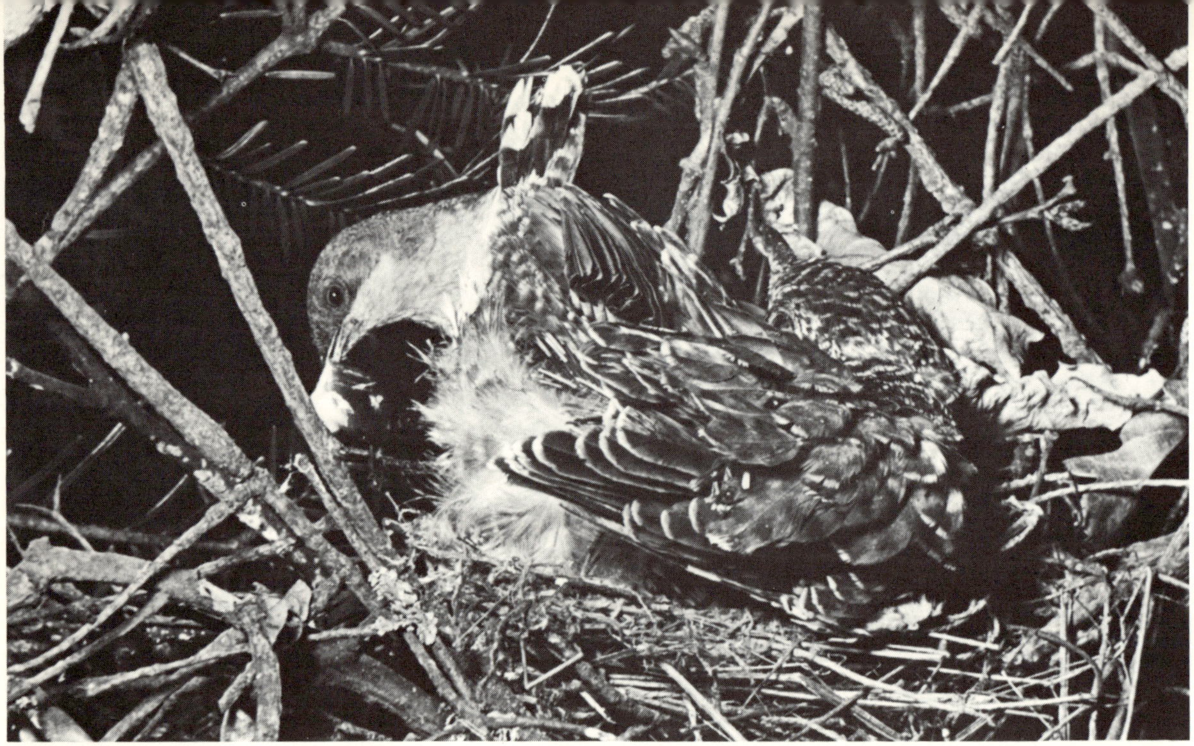

large number of eggs and deposits them in the nests of small birds. Jenner found that the cuckoo's eggs were as small as, if not smaller than, the other eggs, but that they were heavier (*i.e.* 55g. compared to 43g.) The cuckoo mimics the hawk and frightens the foster parents from their nests. With the passage of generations, cuckoos return to the nests of the same type of foster parents and can produce identically coloured eggs.

In June 1786, Jenner was twice able to replace a dislodged hedgesparrow's egg into its nest. He took the young cuckoo out of the nest and the young hedgesparrow was successfully hatched. Later he put the cuckoo back into the nest and the little hedgesparrow was then ejected. Because the foster parents were so alarmed at all this Jenner deduced, wrongly, that hedgesparrows were responsible.

Jenner wrote up his work in the winter of 1786–87 and Hunter presented the paper to the Royal Society on 29th March 1787. Jenner's real discovery

A baby cuckoo demanding food from the parent lesser whitethroat in whose nest the female cuckoo had laid her egg.

A newly hatched cuckoo pushes out an unhatched egg from the nest of its foster-parents.

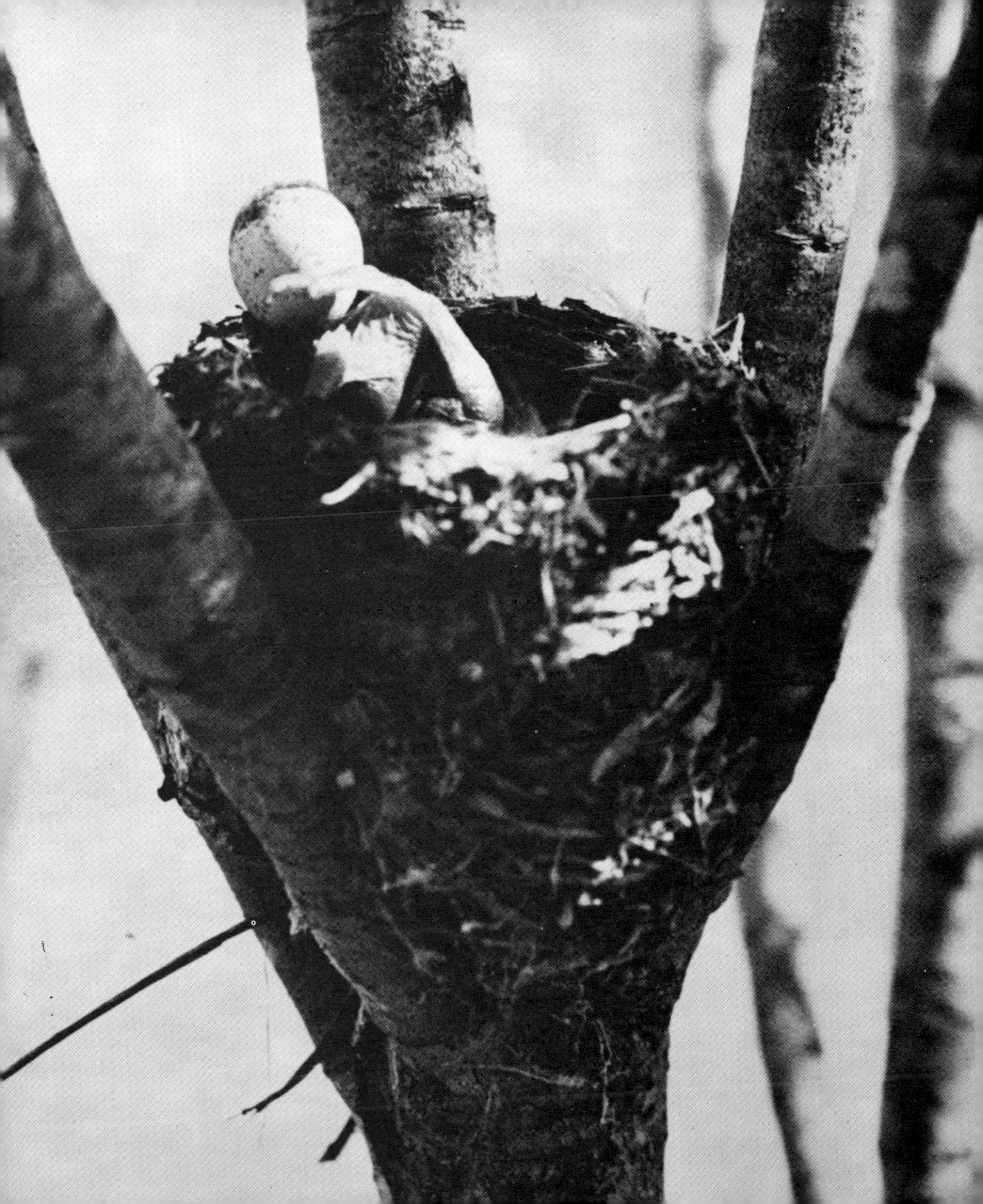

was to come in June 1787. He experimented by putting a young blackbird into a hedgesparrow's nest and there was no ejection, the baby hedgesparrows ending up by sitting on the blackbird's back. He repeated this but the young blackbird smothered the others. On 18th June he was able to watch exactly what happened in a hedgesparrow's nest with one cuckoo in it.

> "The nest was placed so near the extremity of a hedge that I could distinctly see what was going forward in it; and to my astonishment saw the young Cuckoo, though so newly hatched, in the act of turning out the young hedgesparrow.
>
> "The mode of accomplishing this was very curious. The little animal, with the assistance of its rump and wings, contrived to get the bird upon its back, and making a lodgement for the burden by elevating its elbows, clambered backward with it up the side of the nest till it reached the top, where, resting for a moment, it threw off its load with a jerk and quite disengaged it from the nest. It remained in this situation for a short time, feeling about with the extremity of its wings, as if to be convinced whether the business was properly executed, and then dropped into the nest again."

Jenner made his observations again, and experimented by replacing the eggs of the newly-hatched hedgesparrows. He noticed that the cuckoo could only perform the act in the first few days of its life. Thereafter the depression in its back between its wings, into which the object of ejection was allowed to fall, became filled up and the bird was no longer able to displace another egg or bird. Jenner also attached a little lead anchor to a cuckoo's leg, and this foiled it. Later he saw a contest between two cuckoos hatched in the same nest. Eventually one succeeded in turning the other out. Jenner's original paper was amended and read to the Royal Society on 13th March 1788. He was elected Fellow on 26th

February 1789.

As with Jenner's work on vaccination the story of the young cuckoo was greeted with disbelief, scorn and ridicule. Later, the antivaccinationists were to use this to attack Jenner on vaccination—if he was wrong about the cuckoo, so he must be wrong about vaccination! Even eighty years later a well-known naturalist denied that the cuckoo could do this. Gradually Jenner's observations were corroborated, but 140 years were to elapse before the eviction process was photographed in 1929 and shown to the Linnaean Society by F. H. Lancum.

The sequel to the work on the cuckoo, which was put aside during the early years of defending vaccination, was his study of the migration of birds. At that time it was thought that birds which were only seen in the summer either hibernated during the winter or spent the time submerged in ponds or mud. Jenner's observations threw a new light on the matter. He proved that birds could not survive prolonged immersion in water and so could not remain submerged, and that they always arrived in good condition after the winter, unlike animals which hibernated. These facts were coupled with observations made of land birds which could fly across the seas and oceans, even those which were supposedly poor performers in the air. Wild geese shot in Newfoundland were found with maize, from further south, in their crops.

Jenner made another observation during this work, that migratory birds tend to return each year to their previous home. Jenner's main point is that birds migrate to produce offspring, and once that is done they are ready to leave.

Jenner's other interest in natural history included the study of the action of different manures on plants and fruit trees, and the observations on the value of the earthworm (studied in detail later by Darwin) to animal economy in breaking up and aerating the soil.

Jenner's role as an experimental naturalist is often overshadowed by the fame he earned for introducing vaccination to control smallpox; but it is part of the background from which vaccination came. Jenner started his life as a naturalist by making a collection of dormice. He finished it with his work on the migration of birds.

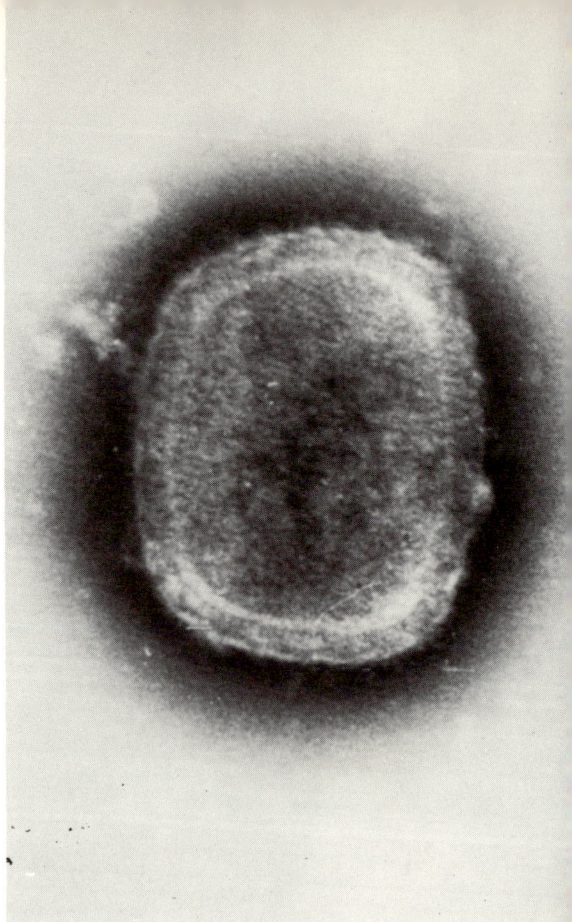

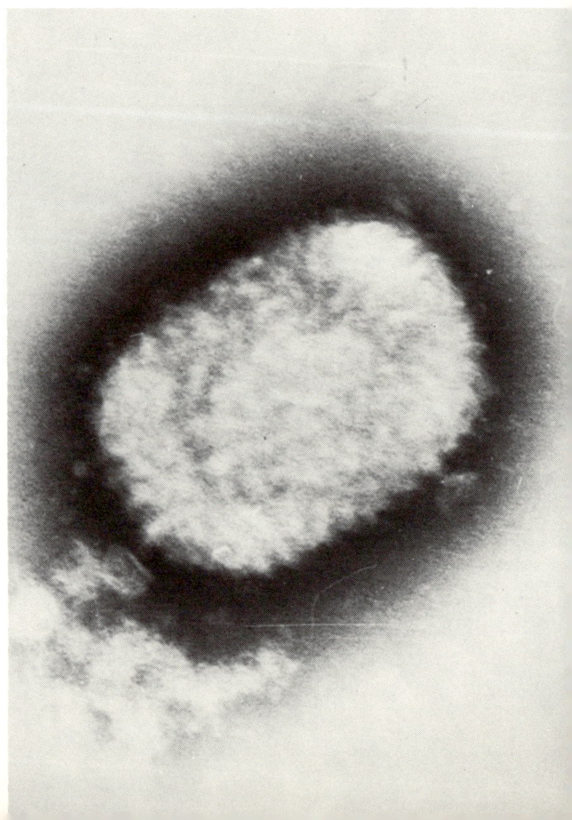

5 *Smallpox*

Smallpox, otherwise known as Variola, is caused by a virus. A virus is the smallest living organism and cannot be seen by the conventional microscope. In 1898 Loeffler found that some living organisms could pass through bacterial filters and these became known as filter-passing ultra-microscopic viruses. With the development of the electron microscope it is now possible to see viruses, and the smallpox virus was observed in 1964 by J. C. N. Westwood. The smallpox virus belongs to a family called the pox viruses (first suspected by Jenner). Unlike bacteria a virus can only survive by entering a living cell and becoming attached to the nucleo-protein. Conventional antibiotics used against bacteria neither inhibit nor destroy viruses. The word "virus" is known to have been used in Elizabethan times when it meant a venom or a poisonous substance. Jenner was one of the first to use it about a disease and since his time it has been adopted as a medical term.

Smallpox, like many other virus diseases, can pass from one person to another, either by direct contact, or by droplet infection from the nose, throat and chest ("coughs and sneezes spread diseases" was an old wartime motto). In addition the disease is spread by handling infected clothing, bedlinen, towels or some article used by the infected person. In such circumstances, these potentially dangerous objects are called fomites. A smallpox epidemic can spread just as quickly as an influenza virus epidemic.

Once inside the body a generalized illness develops over a period of ten to fourteen days (the incubation period). A viraemia occurs when the virus multiplies and circulates in the blood and causes severe general

Opposite Two different types of vaccinia virus magnified 180,000 times.

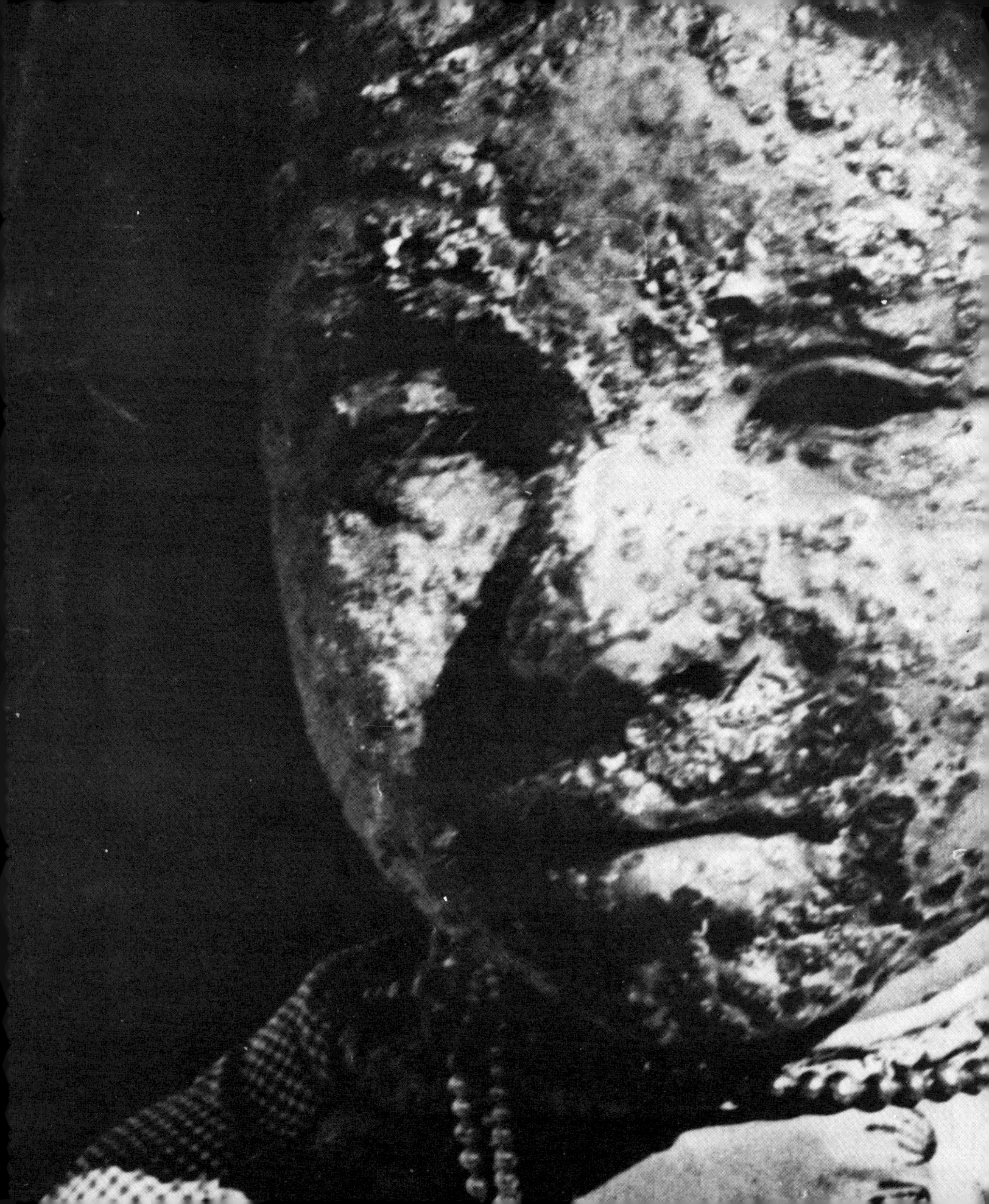

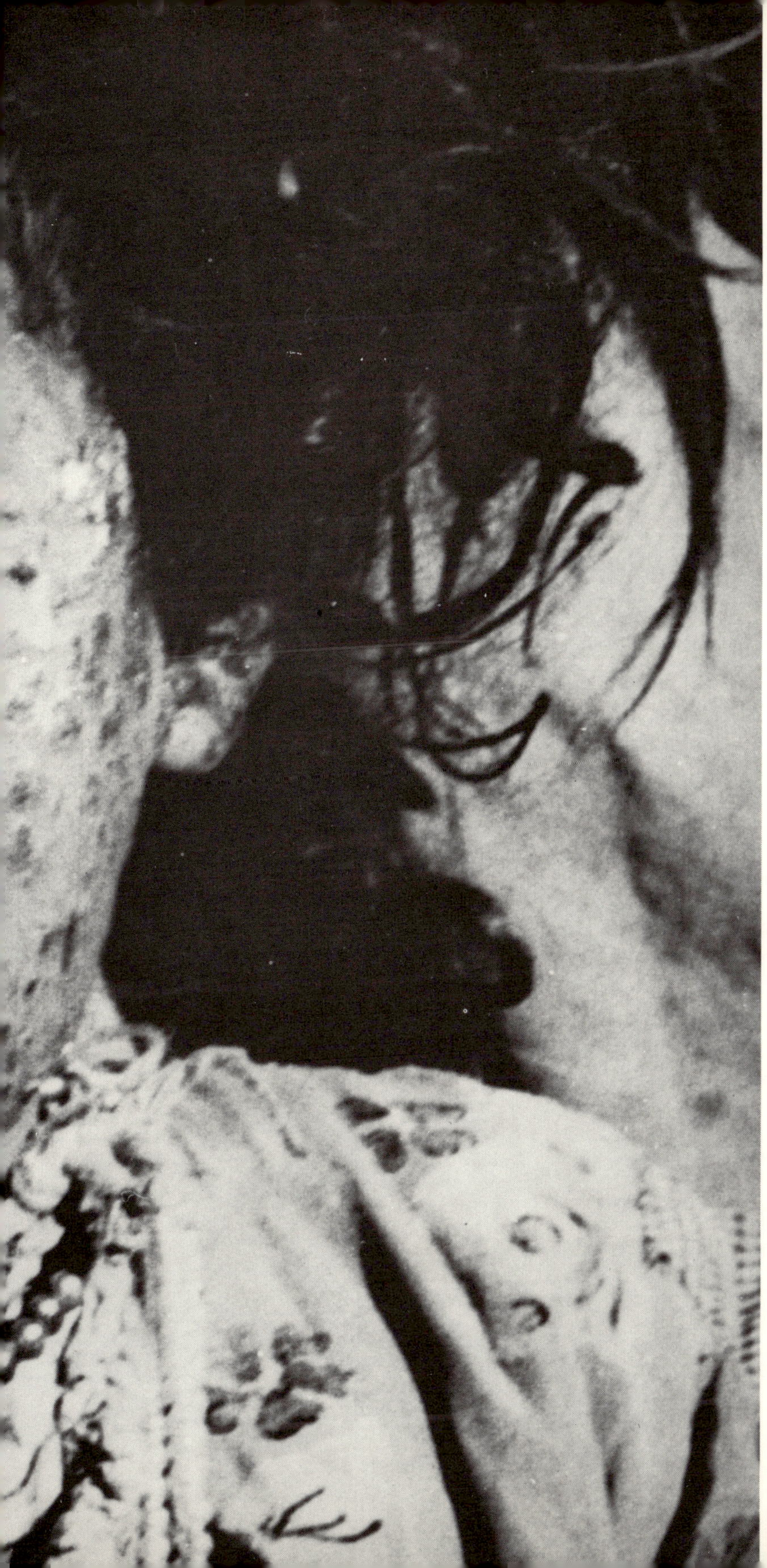

Smallpox still occurs frequently in Afghanistan. Even if this small girl survives the disease she will bear its scars for life.

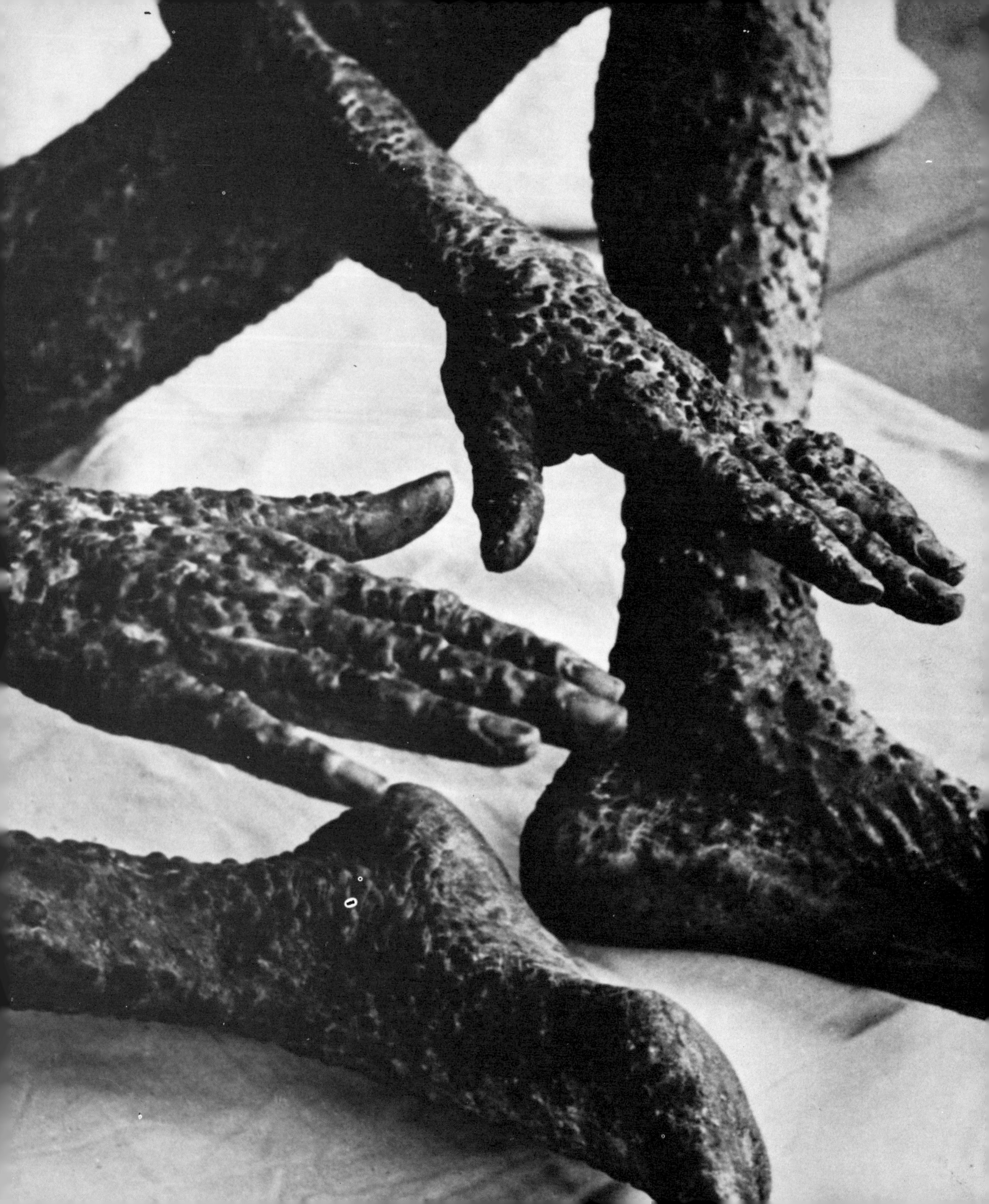

Smallpox pustules covering the arms and legs of a man from the Ivory Coast, West Africa. Smallpox attacks all races of man, no-one is safe unless he has been vaccinated.

effects including a rash which resembles measles. This can lead to confusion in the diagnosis and early recognition of the disease, and at one time smallpox and measles were thought to be related. The pox virus then settles in all the organs of the body including the skin, where it produces itching spots which become blisters (vesicles) and finally pustules. The pustules dry into scabs and these separate to form scars. The disfigurement caused by these scars is made worse by secondary bacterial infection. Apparently, the scarring of King Louis XV was so bad that he seemed to have two noses. In the smallpox victim the exposed parts of the body, face, hands, arms and legs are the main sites for the skin eruptions, as opposed to chickenpox (varicella) in which the eruptions tend to favour the trunk. The mouth, tongue and throat may also be affected in smallpox.

The severity of smallpox varies. In the severest form, bleeding takes place in the skin eruptions and in the internal organs, and death can take place within a few days. Anyone who survives the onslaught of smallpox is liable to die of complications such as pneumonia, heart failure or brain damage. Those recovering may be insane, paralyzed, deaf or subject to painful neuritis, as well as disfigured by the scars, and between 25 and 50 per cent of those who catch severe smallpox will die.

Smallpox has been the scourge of the human race ever since recorded history began. It was present in China and Egypt, where scars have been found on mummies, centuries before Christ. Endemic in the Middle East, the disease was spread by the Crusades. The Spaniards carried it to the American continent where it decimated the Mexican nation by killing as many as three and a half million people. Other voyagers to America caused the death from the disease of half the population of North American Indians. The negro suffered more severely than the white man. Rich and poor alike were at risk.

turn to page 50

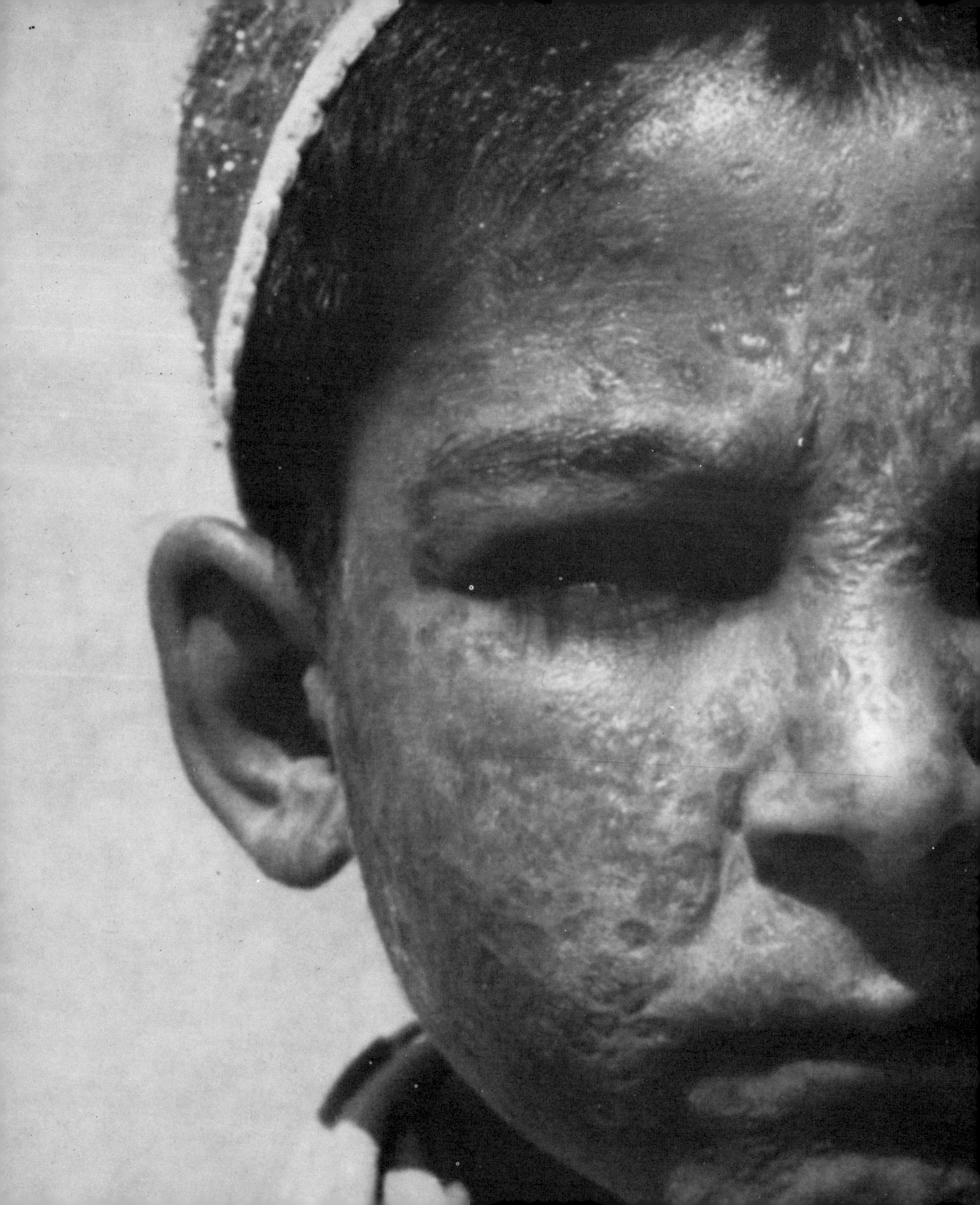

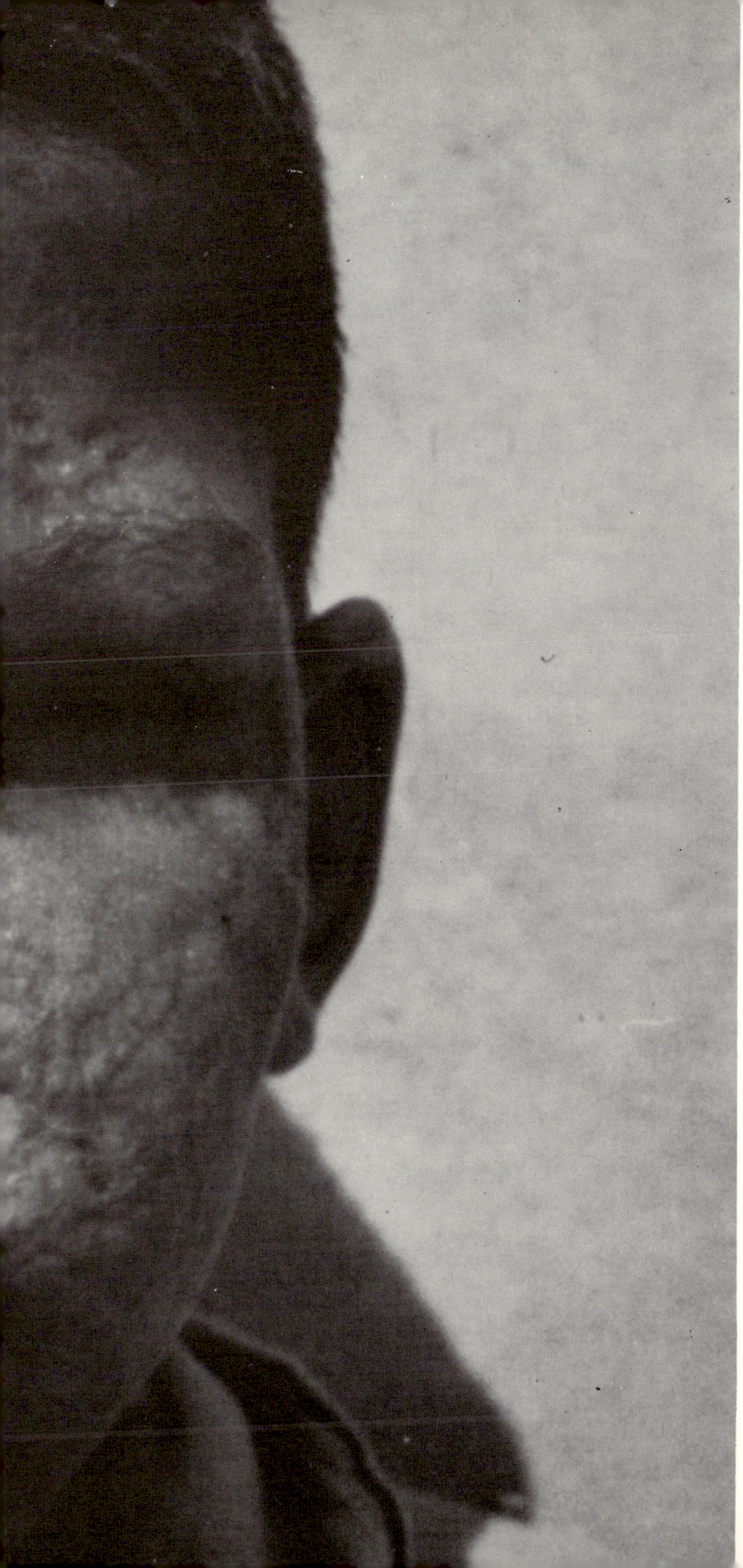

Smallpox was common in England and Europe less than two hundred years ago. Towns and villages were full of people who looked like this Afghan boy. If the disease did not kill them, it scarred them for life.

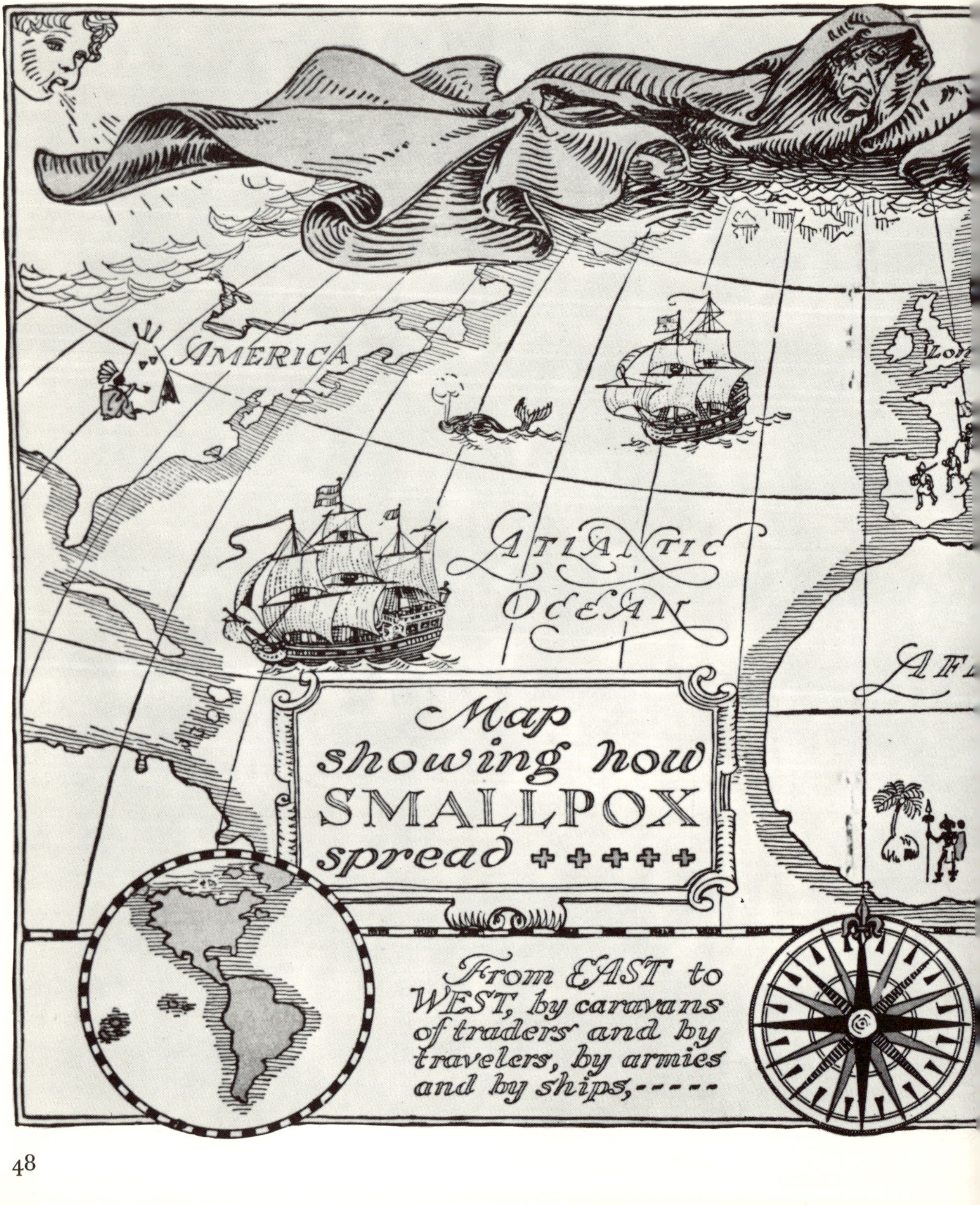
AMERICA
ATLANTIC
OCEAN
Map
showing how
SMALLPOX
spread ✚✚✚✚✚
From EAST to
WEST, by caravans
of traders and by
travelers, by armies
and by ships,-----

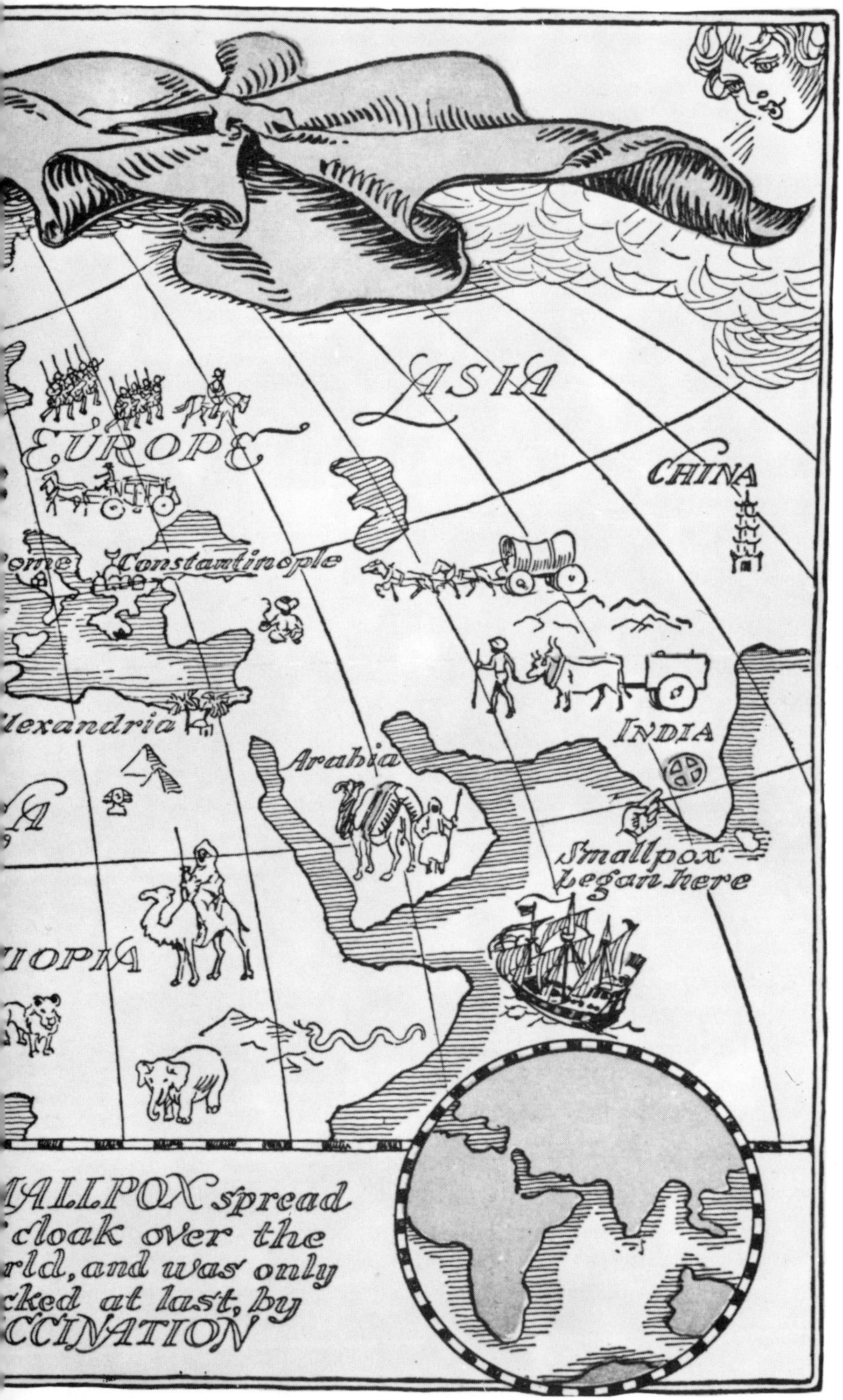

Map showing how smallpox spread across the world from India, where it first began.

c

Among the more illustrious victims were the Roman Emperor Marcus Aurelius, King Louis XV of France, who fell to his second attack, and the English Queen Mary, wife of William of Orange, who died from it in 1694 at the age of 33. London's earliest recorded epidemic was in 1628. It has been said that in the century following Queen Mary's death, during the hundred years before Jenner's introduction of vaccination, sixty million people in Europe died from the disease. Macaulay described this terrifying pestilence in the early eighteenth century in his *History:* "That disease, over which science has since achieved a succession of glorious and beneficent victories, was the most terrible of all the ministers of death. The havoc of the plague had been far more rapid; but plague has visited our shores only once or twice within living memory; and smallpox was always present, filling the churchyard with corpses, tormenting with constant fear all whom it had not yet stricken, leaving on those whose lives were spared, the hideous traces of its power, turning the babe into a changeling at which the mother shuddered, making the eyes and cheeks of the betrothed maiden objects of horror to the lover . . ."

Some thirty or so years before Jenner was born, a method of inoculation was introduced to try and protect individuals from the effects of the disease. This was smallpox inoculation (variolous inoculation or variolation) in which a small amount of matter from a smallpox pustule of a victim was introduced into the skin of a susceptible individual by the scratch of a needle. After an incubation period the inoculated person suffered from a mild attack of smallpox and providing the subject was in good health (as a healthy child, the usual subject, would be) and the virus not particularly virulent, there was a fair chance of survival and a lasting immunity from smallpox. Unfortunately, this practice actually

Opposite Instruments used in China and India for variolation, an early attempt to combat the scourge of smallpox. Dried smallpox scabs were ground into powder which was kept in the container on the right. When a patient was to be treated some of the powder was taken out with the spatula (centre), put into the silver tube (left) and blown into the nose of the patient. It was not effective.

Below Queen Mary, wife of William III of England, died from smallpox in 1694.

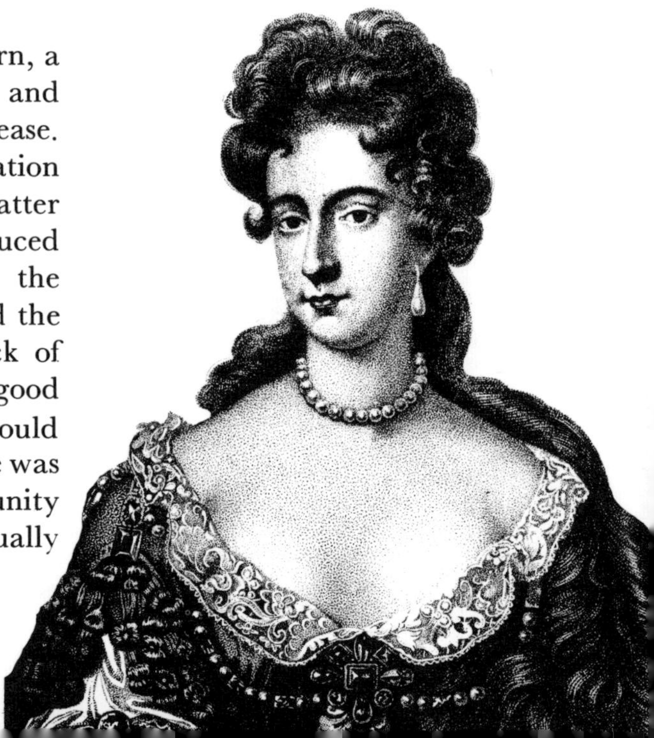

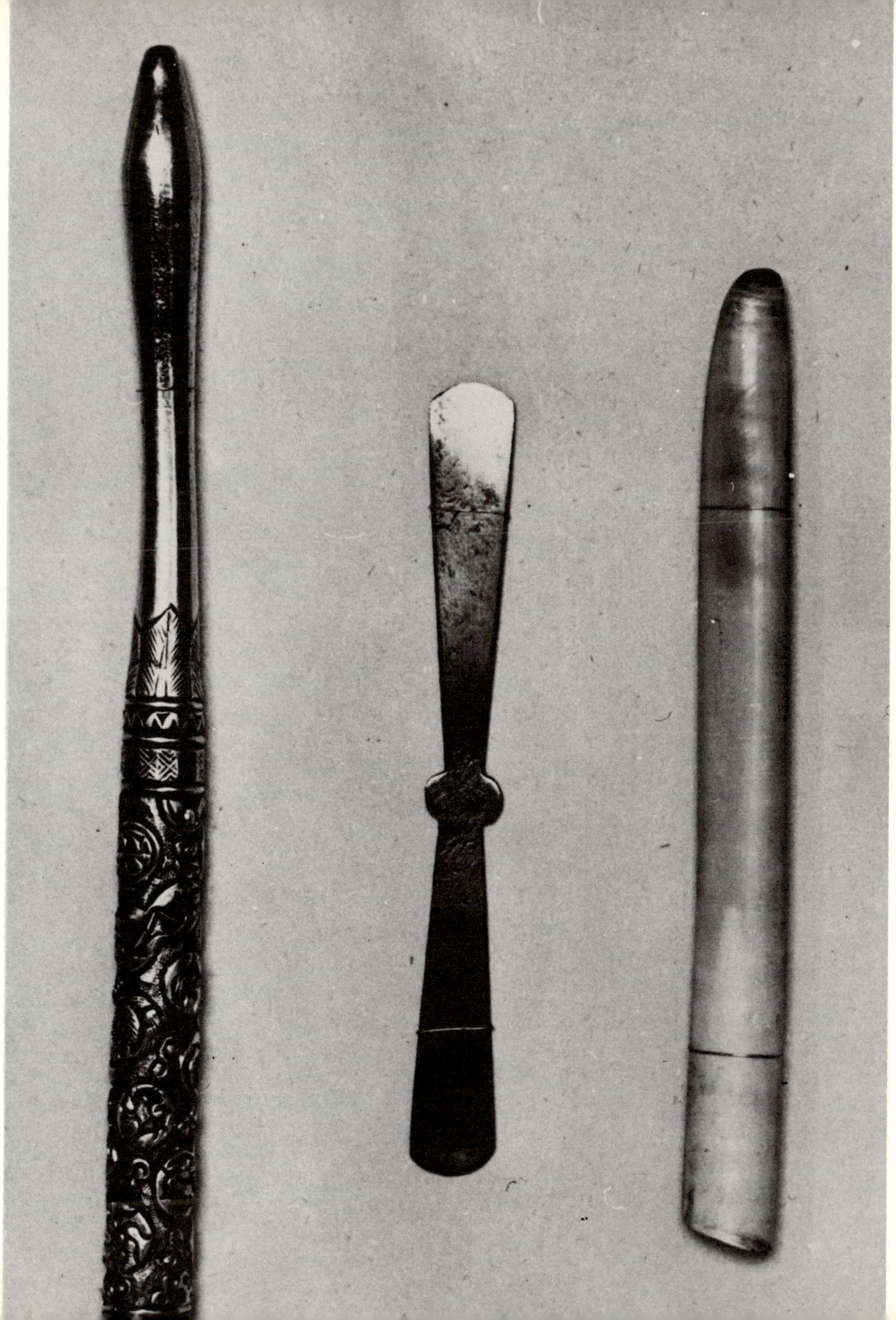

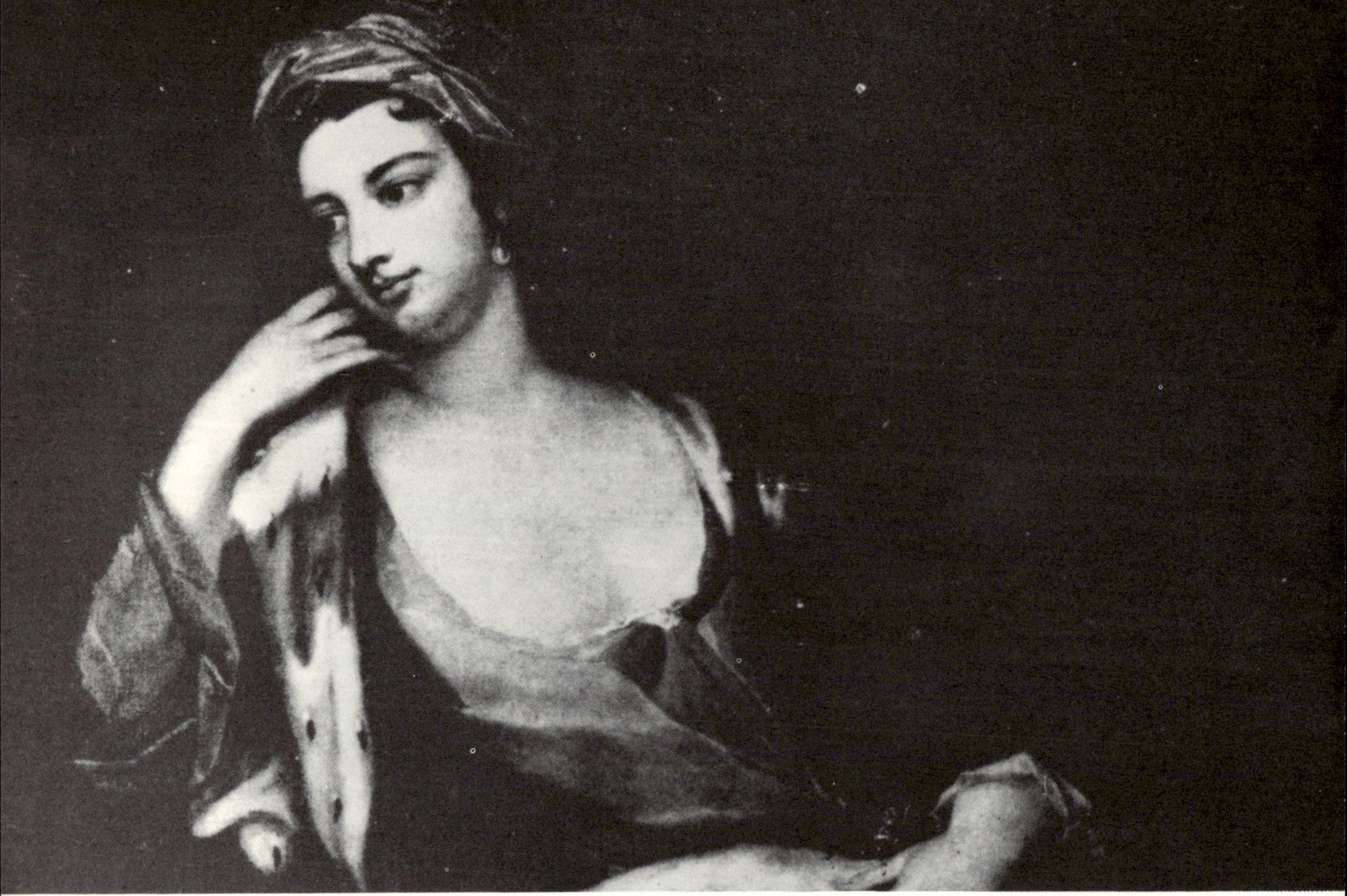

disseminated the disease among the uninoculated, particularly the poor who could not afford the fees being charged. It was still possible to succumb to a second attack, like Louis XV if the immunity wore off.

The practice of smallpox inoculation came from Turkey. It was popularized in England by Lady Mary Wortley Montagu who had lived for a while in Turkey. On 1st April 1717, she wrote from Constantinople to an acquaintance in England and reported how common the method was there. In September of each year when the weather was cooling, old women used to go around inoculating groups of people who wished to have protection with

Lady Mary Wortley Montagu, wife of the British Ambassador to Turkey, observed that inoculation against smallpox was often successfully carried out there. When she returned to England in 1718 she did much to promote inoculation as a means of preventing the disease.

smallpox matter. Lady Montagu reported the technique and the satisfactory results that it seemed to achieve and felt it was her duty to introduce it to England.

Royalty and heads of state, besides being patrons of art and science, often helped to publicize new ideas in medicine, and this happened with smallpox inoculation. It was during one of the frequent epidemics of smallpox, in 1721–22, that Lady Montagu persuaded Princess Caroline to have her children inoculated. King George I ordered the inoculation of six condemned men in Newgate prison. Five of them contracted the disease and survived, and the sixth, who had not mentioned that he had had smallpox before, also survived. All six were freed. Then eleven charity children were inoculated successfully by Claudius Amyand, master of the Barber Surgeons Company and sergeant surgeon to the King. Amyand then successfully inoculated the two young Princesses, Caroline and Amelia. All this was followed by a great demand for smallpox inoculation and various exponents of the method immediately appeared. Thomas Dimsdale received a fee of £10,000, a pension of £500 and a barony for successfully inoculating Empress Catherine the Great of Russia. The Suttons developed their own technique, making the scratch wound as small as possible, and in addition to inoculating over 2,500 people, sold their secret to other practitioners.

When Jenner was a boy he too was inoculated with smallpox. The procedure was described by Fosbroke: "He was a fine ruddy boy, and, at eight years of age, was, with many others, put under a preparatory process for inoculation with the smallpox. This preparation lasted six weeks. He was bled to ascertain whether his blood was fine; was purged repeatedly, till he became emaciated and feeble; was kept on a very low diet . . . After this barbarism of human veterinary practice, he was removed to one of the usual inoculation stables, and haltered up with the others, in a terrible state of disease."

Apparently Jenner's recovery from this ordeal was slow, and complicated by insomnia and noises in the head. He became unduly sensitive to sudden sharp noises, a tendency which distressed him very much in later years. His experience of the method was something he was never to forget.

As the eighteenth century progressed, the smallpox grew worse in spite of inoculation. The passage (pronounced "passarge") from person to person caused an increase in the virulence of the virus and so inoculation itself was spreading the disease. In the second half of the century the Bills of Mortality showed a later Royal Commission on Vaccination (1896) that in England one in ten people died from smallpox in the second half of the eighteenth century, compared with one in fourteen in the first half. By 1762, long before Jenner's work on vaccination, smallpox was increasing so fast in France that inoculation became illegal. England could not or would not make up her mind until 1840 possibly because of vested interests, an intense anti-vaccine lobby, envy, and disbelief that a country surgeon and naturalist who observed cuckoos could possibly be right.

6 *Cow Pox and Vaccination*

At the time of Jenner's observations and experiments with cow pox there was no knowledge of the actual cause or nature of infective diseases, whether due to bacteria or viruses. About 100 years were to elapse until Louis Pasteur demonstrated by fermentation experiments that infections were not caused by "spontaneous generation." This work met with disbelief, resistance, ridicule and even riots.

Later Joseph Lister was also taunted for his work on antisepsis and germs. "Show us these germs," his opponents insisted. But this was not possible, for the staining of bacteria to make them visible and their identification had to wait for Paul Ehrlich, working with anilene dyes. While the body of knowledge about infectious diseases was so small even in the nineteenth century, the ignorance was, if possible, greater, in Jenner's time. Jenner, as already recounted, used the word "virus" about smallpox only because this was the word then used to describe a poison or venom.

The format of Jenner's thesis on Cow Pox (called *The Inquiry*), undoubtedly the result of the training he received at the hand of John Hunter, is much the same as that needed for a medical thesis of today. It includes an introduction, a statement of the clinical problem, a review of existing knowledge (nowadays this becomes a review of the literature), the presentation of an hypothesis, a description and critical evaluation of methods and experiments, the presentation and discussion of results, and the conclusions.

As a medical practitioner trained in London, Jenner well knew how big the national smallpox problem was. He had, in his childhood, endured the

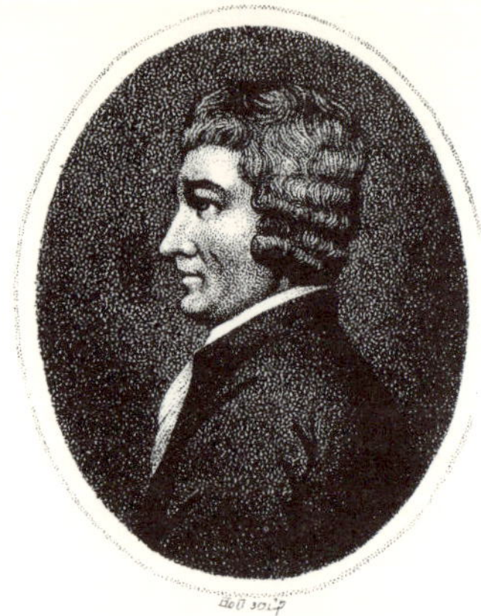

Left Dr. John Lettsom, a well-known physician, who was a staunch supporter of Jenner's ideas about vaccination.

DR. LETTSOM.

JOHN COAKLEY LETTSOM was one of twins, born in December 1741, in Van Dyke Island, near Tortola, within the verge of the tropics. At the age of six years he was sent to England for his education, and was placed under the protection of Mr. Fothergill, a preacher in the Society of Friends, and brother to the celebrated Dr. John Fothergill. By the former, young Lettsom was entrusted to the care of Dr. Sutcliff, to whom he was apprenticed. He was afterwards entered at St. Thomas's hospital, where he acquired those habits of industry, by which the whole of his after life was strongly characterized. He remained there two years, and then returned to his native country, in order to take possession of the property, which had fallen to him by the death of his father and elder brother. This property, however, consisted of very little, besides a number of slaves; whom, to his eternal honour, he immediately emancipated.

Having thus left himself in a manner destitute, he settled for a short time at Tortola as a medical practitioner, and soon established a very respectable practice. He afterwards visited the universities of Edinburgh and Leyden; at the latter, he took the degree of M.D. From Leyden he again came to London, where he commenced practice under the patronage of Dr. Fothergill. The same year, he was admitted a licentiate of the Royal College of Physicians: the year following, elected F.S.A. and, the year after, F.R.S. and very soon afterwards F.L.S.

His popularity, as a friend to science, and still more so as a philanthropist, now rapidly advanced. His subsequent marriage with a very amiable lady, who brought him a considerable fortune, gave him additional opportunities of exercising those feelings of benevolence towards his fellow creatures in distress, which had long glowed in his bosom. His correspondence with persons of the first eminence, both in Europe and America, extended to almost every name there recorded in the annals of science, literature, and benevolence. Dr. Lettsom belonged to almost every literary institution in the world: he was a member of no less than sixteen universities: a fellow of the Royal College of Physicians, Edinburgh; and of nearly every other medical society in England and America. He was treasurer and one of the founders of the Royal Humane Society, and vice-president of the London Philosophical Society; in which honourable chair he was succeeded by his Royal Highness the Duke of Suffolk.

Of the writings of Dr. Lettsom it is impossible here to give even a list; they embrace a variety of interesting topics, every one of them tending to promote the great ends of science or universal benevolence. His last little work was a pamphlet, entitled "Recollections of Dr. Rush." It was written but a few weeks prior to his death. The manuscript was put into the hands of the writer of this, with a modest request, that he might not be "permitted to disgrace himself as an author in his old age." Those who have read the pamphlet will not need to be informed that Dr. Lettsom's powers had suffered nothing by age. This worthy and celebrated physician died after a short illness, on Wednesday, the 1st of November 1815; and his remains were interred in the Friends' burial ground, Little Coleman-street, Bunhill-row. The real value of Dr. Lettsom's character was known only to those who had constant opportunities of viewing him both in public and private life. Though, by artful and designing individuals, he was brought into considerable pecuniary embarrassments towards the close of his days; yet the general tenor of his life was governed by the principles of honour and integrity. The "Life and Correspondence of Dr. Lettsom" have been published in three 8vo vols. by Mr. Pettigrew, who has done ample justice to the numerous merits of his friend.

11

existing preventive method from which he carried the scars on his skin and in his brain and mind. He knew that the disease was being spread by inoculation. Only the death registers, called Bills of Mortality, which were published throughout the country, gave an idea of the prevalence of the current mortal diseases. According to Dr Lettsom, a physician of renown and a firm supporter of Jenner, more than 36,000 people died from smallpox every year, out of a population of twelve millions in Great Britain and Ireland. In Greater London, with a population of one million, eight people died from smallpox every day.

Jenner's hypothesis originated about 1765, when an incident occurred which became firmly imprinted in his mind. A dairymaid attended for an infection of her hand. Having already learned the importance of listening to the detailed history of a complaint, he was struck by her remark that her skin condition could not be smallpox—"I cannot take smallpox for I have had cow pox." Also at that time a short ballad, now well known as a nursery rhyme, was in vogue:

" 'Where are you going to my pretty maid?'
" 'I'm going a milking, Sir,' she said
" 'What is your fortune my pretty maid?'
" 'My face is my fortune, Sir,' she said."

Milkmaids did not have pock-marked and disfigured faces.

During his years with John Hunter, Jenner must have discussed this matter many times. He continually raised the matter for discussion at the medical societies to which he belonged. Apparently Jenner's colleagues threatened to expel him from one of these societies if he continued to harp on the subject!

Jenner realized that the conflicting evidence could only be sorted out by first defining what was true cow pox, and what was not. This he could only do by careful observations and making records

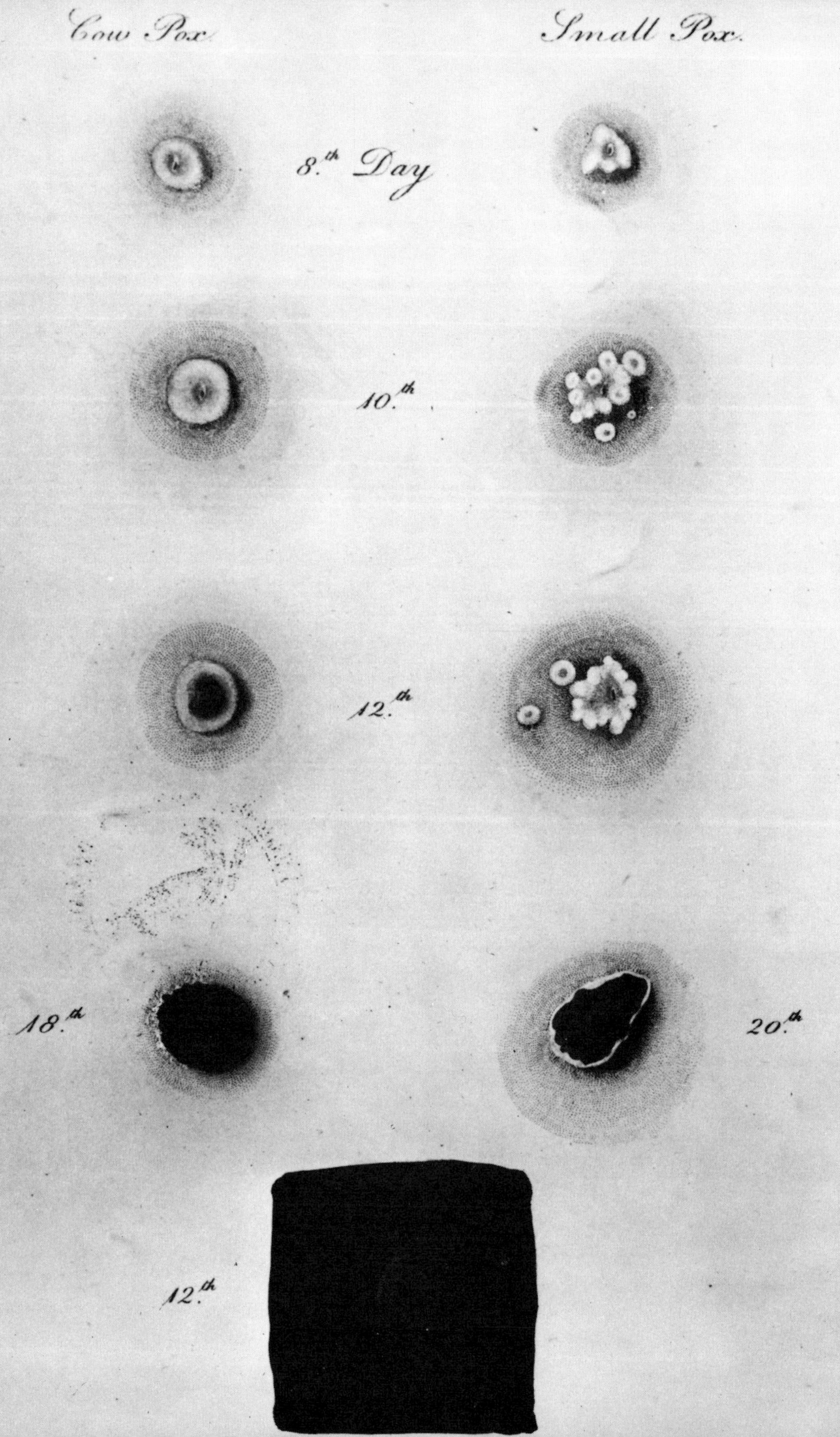

Cow Pox
Small Pox
8.th Day
10.th
12.th
18.th
20.th
12.th

Opposite Drawings made by Jenner of his observations of the differences betaeen cow pox and smallpox pustules on human skin. On the left are the cow pox pustules, on the right those made by smallpox.
Below Jenner's drawing of cow pox pustules on the hand of the dairymaid Sarah Nelmes

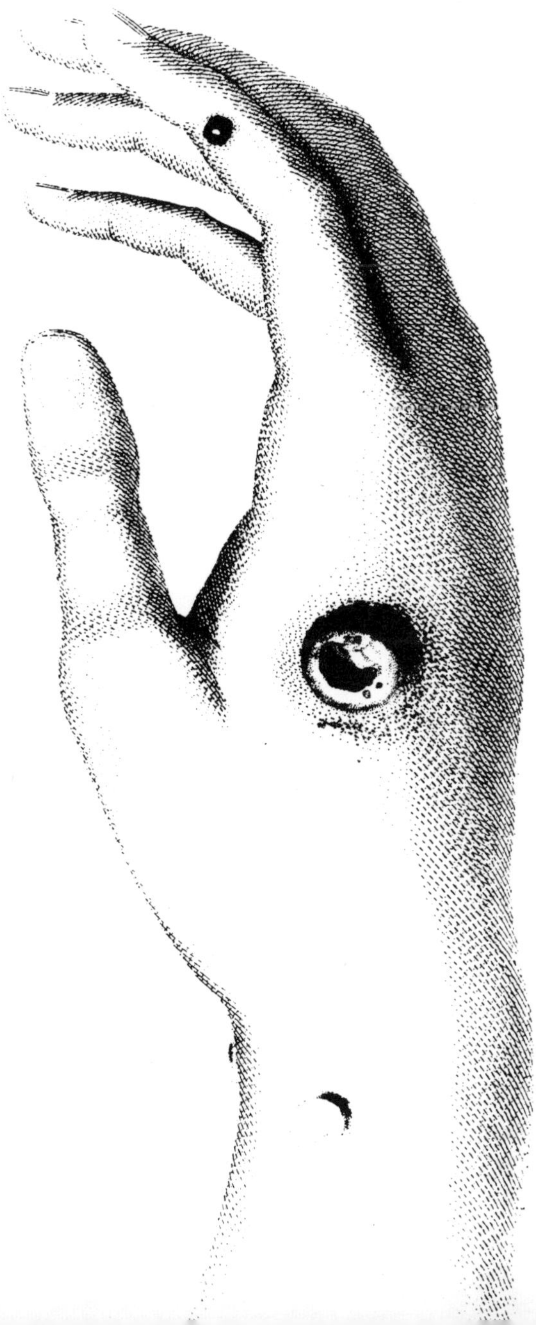

by drawings. Jenner soon realized that cows and milkmaids were liable to suffer from several different kinds of skin eruptions, quite unrelated to cow pox. He was also interested in and puzzled by a skin eruption on horses' heels called "grease." There was some evidence that this, or one form of it, could be passed to cows and from them to milkmaids.

Time passed. His friends were bored with the subject, he became involved with the work on the cuckoo, and he got married and started a family. When he returned to the subject, he knew that the time had come to stop thinking and to try the experiment, but there was then no cow pox available. He inoculated his baby Edward with swine pox, which resulted in some pustules, but this was not a real test. In 1791 a milker who supposedly had had cow pox in the past caught smallpox and this also threatened Jenner's hypothesis, but he deduced that factors such as alterations in virulence and extraneous influences could interfere with the production of immunity.

Jenner wrote: "There were not wanting instances to prove that when the cow pox broke out among the cattle at a dairy, a person who had milked an infected animal and had thereby apparently gone through the disease in common with others, was liable to receive the smallpox afterwards. This . . . gave a painful check to my fond and aspiring hopes: but . . . I resumed my labour with redoubled ardour. The result was fortunate; for I now discovered that the virus of cow pox was liable to undergo progressive changes . . . and that when it was applied to the human skin in its degenerated state it would produce the ulcerative effects in as great a degree as when it was not decomposed, and sometimes far greater, but having lost its specific properties, it was incapable of producing that change upon the human frame which is requisite to render it unsusceptible of variolous contagion: so that it became evident a person might milk a cow one day, and having caught the disease, be for ever secure, while another person milking the same cow the next day might feel the influence of the virus in such a way as to produce a sore or sores . . . yet, as has been observed, the specific quality being lost . . . ."

In support of his idea that an attack of cow pox could prevent smallpox, and also to show that long-lasting immunity was possible, Jenner collected evidence in a series of cases. For example, Joseph Merret had cow pox in 1770. Jenner inoculated him with smallpox in 1795 and it had no effect on him, nor did the smallpox which afflicted his whole family. But might Joseph have had smallpox many years before? Jenner's answer was, in effect, that in a village everybody knew everyone else's business and that records were kept. The second example was Sarah Portlock who had cow pox twenty-seven years before her negative result to smallpox inoculation. Another example was John Phillips, who had had cow pox when he was nine. At the age of fifty-two he was inoculated, without effect, with virulent smallpox. Mary Barge could even nurse smallpox patients without catching the disease because she had had cow pox thirty-one years before. Jenner cites twelve cases, and three others who had immunity after "grease" (horse pox).

In May 1796, Jenner decided to "try the experiment." Case 16 was Sarah Nelmes, a dairymaid . . . "[who] was infected with cow pox from her master's cows . . . received the infection on a part of the hand which had been previously injured by a scratch from a thorn. A large pustulous sore and the usual symptoms accompanying the disease were produced in consequence."

Case 17, 14th May 1796, was James Phipps: "The more accurately to observe the progress of the infection, I selected a healthy boy, about eight years old, for the purpose of inoculation for the cow pox.

Statue commemorating Edward Jenner's vaccination of James Phipps. The importance of this operation to the world's health cannot be overestimated.

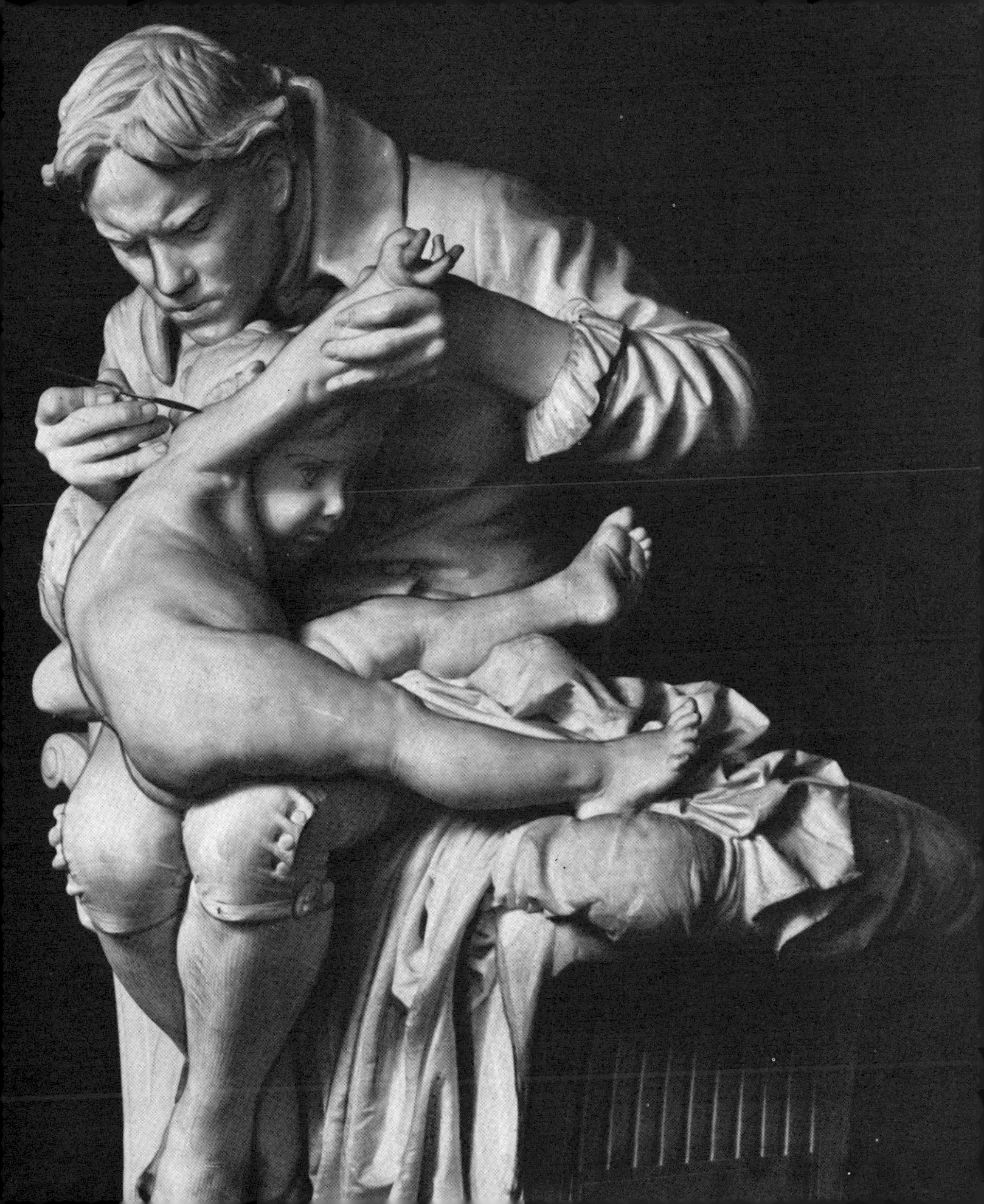

The matter was taken from the sore on the hand of the dairymaid [Sarah Nelmes] . . . and it was inserted, on the 14th May 1796, into the arm of the boy by means of two superficial incisions, barely penetrating the cutis, each about half an inch long . . . On the seventh day he complained of uneasiness in the axilla, and on the ninth he became a little chilly, lost his appetite and had a slight headache. During the whole of this day he was perceptibly indisposed, and spent the night with some degree of restlessness, but on the day following he was perfectly well."

On 19th July 1796, Jenner wrote this historic letter to his friend Edward Gardner:

> "Dear Gardner,
>
> As I promised to let you know how I proceeded in my Inquiry into the nature of that singular disease the Cow Pox being fully satisfied how much you feel interested in its success, you will be gratified in hearing that I have at length accomplished what I have been so long waiting for, the passing of the vaccine virus from one human being to another by the ordinary mode of Inoculation. A Boy of the name of Phipps was inoculated in the arm from a Pustule on the hand of a young woman who was infected by her Master's cows. Having never seen the disease but in its casual way before, that is, when communicated from the cow to the hand of the Milker, I was astonished at the close resemblance of the Pustules in some of their stages to the variolous pustules. But now listen to the most delightful part of my story. The boy has since been inoculated for the Smallpox which as I ventured to predict, produced no effect. I shall now pursue my Experiments with redoubled ardour. Believe me.
>
> Yours very sincerely,
> Edwd. Jenner.
>
> 19th July 1796—Berkeley."

The first page of Jenner's letter to his friend Edward Gardner, mentioned in the text on the left.

July 19. 1796 Highly interesting containing an account of the inoculation of Phipps

(6)

Dear Gardner

As I promised to let you know
how I proceeded in my Enquiry into the
nature of that singular disease the Cow Pox
& being fully satisfied how much you feel interested
in its success, you will be gratified in hearing
that I have at length accomplish'd what
I have been so long waiting for, the passing of
the vaccine Virus from one human being
to another by the ordinary mode of Inoculation.
A Boy of the name of Phipps was inoc-
-culated in the Arm from a Pustule on the
hand of a young Woman who was infected
by her Masters Cows. Having never seen
the disease but in its casual way before,

Jenner's ardour was frustrated by the disappearance of cow pox from Berkeley and it was not until February 1798 that a mare developed sore heels, and cows on the same farm followed with cow pox. Three men on the farm caught cow pox; Jenner seized his chance. He inoculated a boy from one of the cows and then passed the cow pox from this to another boy, and so to several children and adults, and so on.

Jenner wrote up his thesis firstly in two draft manuscripts. It was printed and published in 1798 as a pamphlet entitled *An Inquiry into the causes and effects of the Variolae Vaccinae, a disease discovered in some of the western counties of England, particularly Gloucestershire, and known by the name of the Cow Pox* by Edward Jenner, M.D., F.R.S. & c.

Corrections and additions were made in two later editions, the second in 1800 and the third in 1801. It was translated into several languages and was often reprinted—particularly during the nineteenth century smallpox epidemics.

What became of James Phipps? Jenner used him to demonstrate smallpox immunity and inoculated him twenty times without smallpox appearing. Phipps lived to enjoy his old age. Jenner built a cottage for him near the Chantry and opposite the church. It is now the Jenner Museum. The cow that infected Sarah Nelmes was called Blossom, and was allowed to end her days in the pastures at Berkeley.

7 *Vaccination Grows in Britain*

The reception of a new idea has been compared with the reaction of the human body (the production of of antibodies) to a bacterial or viral substance (antigen). Pasteur and Lister, also encountered much hostility to their discoveries. They often found that their main critics were men of standing in their profession who could not take the trouble to follow accurately the original descriptions of the methods involved in a discovery. Faraday and Sir James Simpson received the same treatment. Even in the 1930s a popular song voiced such an attitude to other pioneers such as Edison and the Wright brothers. Jenner had to face this problem long before all of them.

Immediately before the publication of *The Inquiry into Cow Pox* in 1798 Jenner travelled to London, hoping to be in immediate demand to show his new method. Nothing happened. No one came to see him. No one seemed interested. After three months, disappointed, Jenner went home to Berkeley, but before doing so he left a quill of dried cow pox matter (lymph) with one of John Hunter's old pupils, Mr Cline, a surgeon to St. Thomas's Hospital. Mr Cline, who was not particularly interested in cow pox, had among his patients a boy suffering from a diseased hip on whom he was going to try a method of treatment called counter-irritation. This method, still in use today, involves applying an irritant to the area of skin which has a similar nerve supply to the affected joint and surrounding muscles, so giving reflex relief from pain in the joint and from muscle spasms. Cline decided to try the lymph as a counter-irritant. He punctured the skin twice over the hip joint, and applied the lymph. At the beginning of

August Jenner received a letter.

Lincoln's Inn Fields, 2d. Aug. 1798.

"The cow pox experiment has succeeded admirably. The child sickened on the seventh day; and the fever, which was moderate, subsided on the eleventh day. The inflammation extended to about four inches diameter and then gradually subsided . . . I have since inoculated him with smallpox matter in three places, which were slightly inflamed on the third day, and then subsided.

"Dr Lister, who was formerly physician to the Smallpox Hospital, attended the child with me, and he is convinced that it is not possible to give him the smallpox.

"I think the substituting of cow pox poison for the smallpox promises to be one of the greatest improvements that has ever been made in medicine; for it is not only so safe in itself, but also does not endanger others by contagion, in which way the smallpox has done infinite mischief. The more I think on the subject the more I am impressed with its importance. With great esteem I am, dear Sir,

Your faithful servant, Henry Cline."

This was all that was needed to set cow pox inoculation going. Within six weeks after the publication of *The Inquiry* cow pox had become the talk of London's medical and social world. However, it took ten years for the practice to become accepted generally, and for Jenner these were ten hard years of contending with antagonistic physicians and surgeons and with the general misunderstanding about the recognition of true cow pox and the technique required. He had to cope with the snubs, the public ridicule, the claims of prior discovery, the setting up of enquiries, and the fortunes of various vaccine institutes.

Among the medical antagonists the first was the physician to the Empress of Austria, a Dr Ingenhouse,

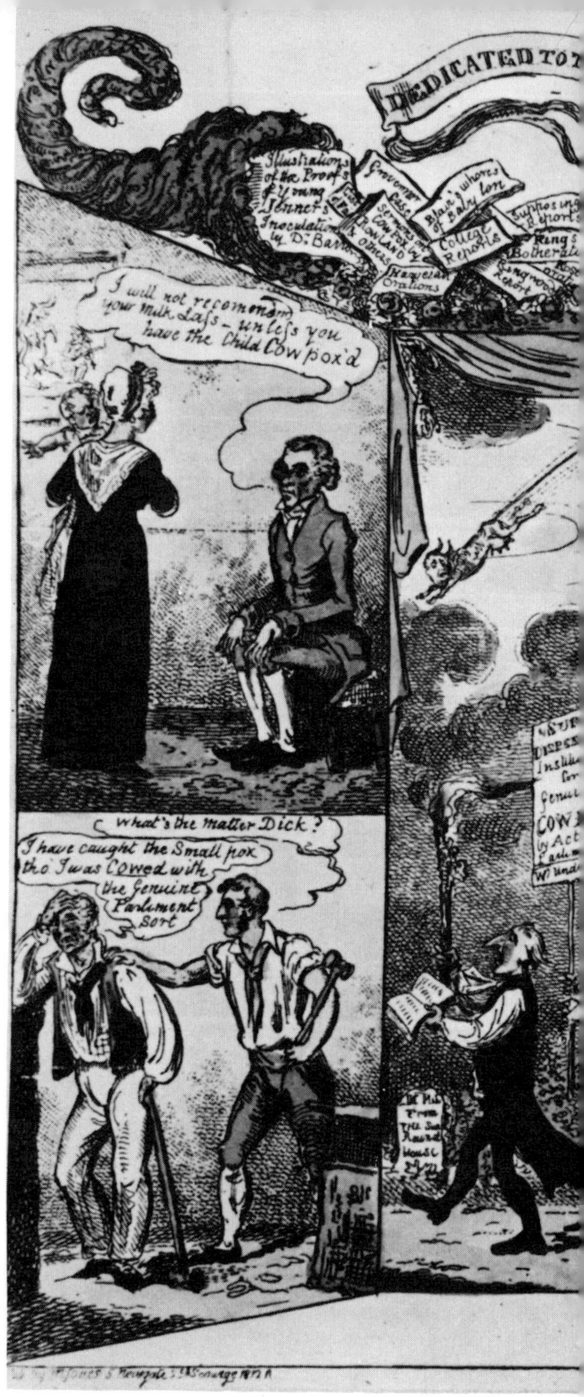

I will not recomend your Milk Lass - unless you have the Child Cow pox'd
What's the matter Dick?
I have caught the Small pox tho' I was Cowed with the Genuine Parliment Sort

Jenner had to put up with much opposition to his ideas. The medical profession opposed him, and even popular cartoonists like George Cruikshank drew cartoons ridiculing his work.

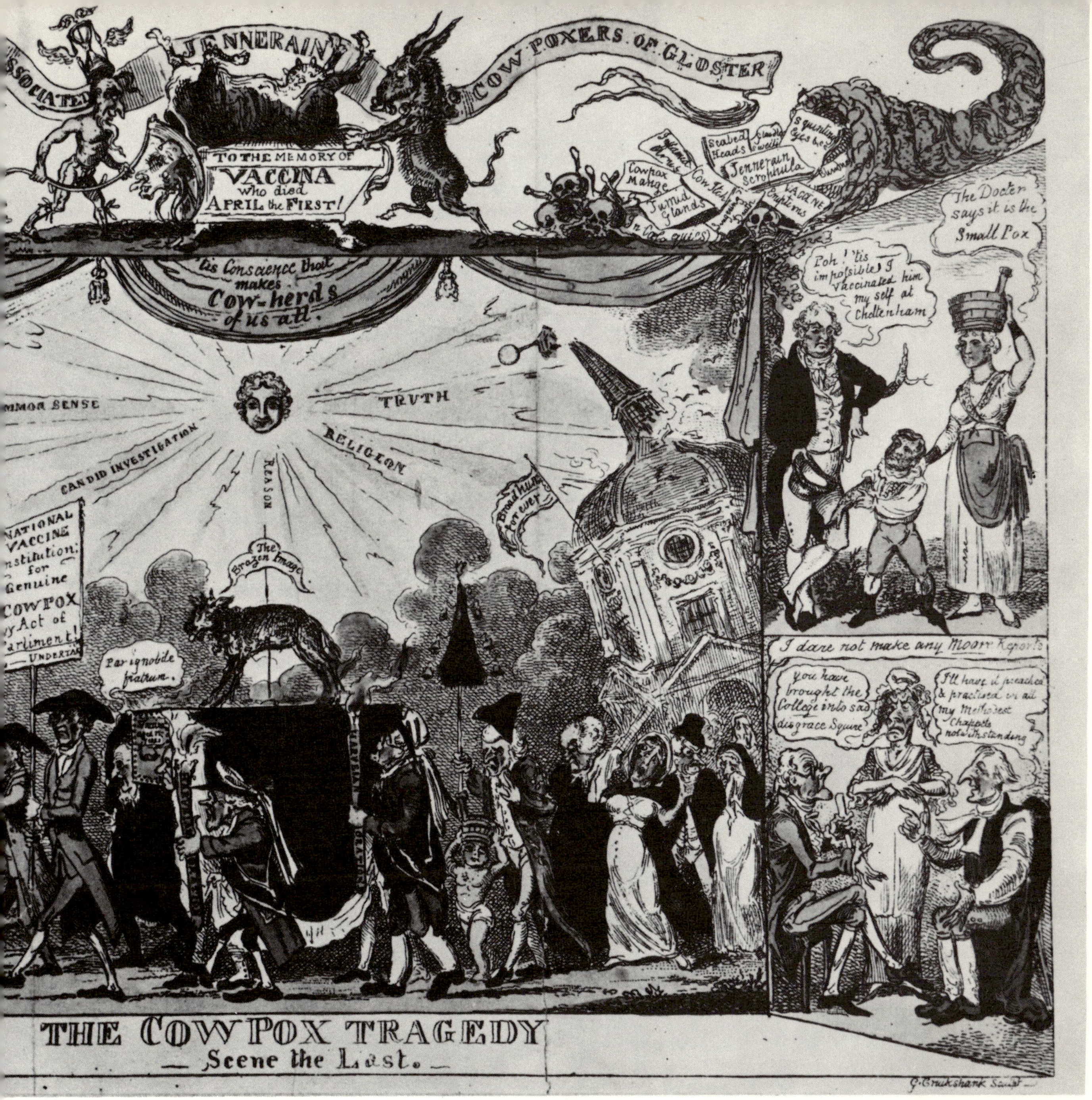
ASSOCIATED
JENNERAIN
COW POXERS OF GLOSTER
TO THE MEMORY OF
VACCINA
who died
APRIL the FIRST!
Cowpox Mange
Scabed Heads
Jennerain Scrophula
Tumid Glands
'tis Conscience that makes Cow-herds of us all.
TRUTH
RELIGION
REASON
CANDID INVESTIGATION
The Brazen Image
Broadhurst for ever
Par ignobile fratrum.
The Doctor says it is the Small Pox
Poh! 'tis impossible! I vaccinated him my self at Cheltenham
I dare not make any Moore Reports
You have brought the College into sad disgrace Squire
I'll have it preached & practised in all my Methodist Chappels notwithstanding
THE COWPOX TRAGEDY
Scene the Last.
G. Cruikshank Sculpt

who happened to be visiting England. He based his attack on the report of one farmer who said he had contracted smallpox after a previous infection with cow pox. Neither farmer nor physician could identify or define true cow pox.

It was Dr Pearson of St. George's Hospital who gave Jenner the most anxiety, however, because he seemed to want to take the whole thing over and set himself up as discoverer and supplier of cow pox lymph. He, with others, decided to set up a vaccine board in order to promote the business. Jenner was left off this board, but was later offered the title of extra Consulting Physician on, so it is said, payment of one guinea as an annual subscription!

Dr Pearson inoculated fourteen people on an estate in Sussex. All became gravely ill and one died. Jenner guessed why: if the true cow pox on a donor had not been identified, the wrong lymph could have been used. Later Jenner gave the owner of the estate some pure cow pox lymph from Gloucestershire, and personally vaccinated two hundred people successfully. Dr Pearson opposed Jenner's cause at the first parliamentary enquiry by producing the doubtful claims of others to have discovered vaccination. When the Medical Society of London proposed the award of a gold medal to Jenner, Dr Pearson opposed this, unsuccessfully, saying that Jenner's work was "no discovery" and "a rascally ignorant business."

There was trouble, too, with Dr Woodville, physician to the Smallpox Hospital. Cow pox was found among some cows in Grays Inn Road (now in the centre of London). Dr Woodville made a trial inoculation at his hospital, but again cow pox became confused with smallpox, the patients were mixed up and records were not kept. Later, Dr Woodville admitted to the House of Commons committee that he could not be sure of his observations. Later, he was to vaccinate correctly and successfully.

Dr Moseley was one of the opponents who ridiculed the new discovery. He argued that if people were inoculated with cow pox they would show bestial characteristics. This ridicule prompted

One doctor even claimed that people would come to look like animals if inoculated with cowpox, an idea satirised by this cartoon.

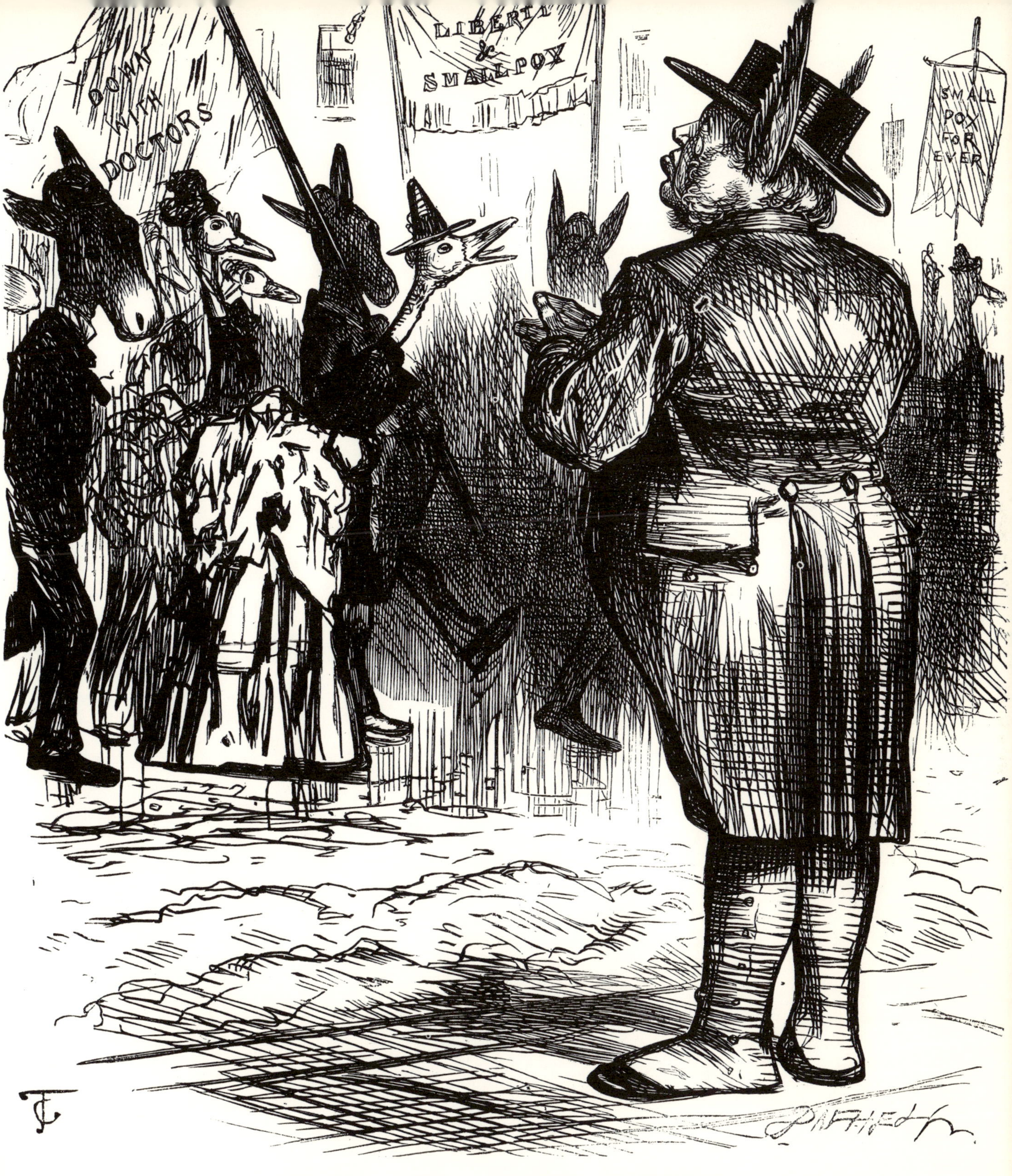

JACK OF BOTH SIDES;

SYMPATHETIC, BUT DOUBTFUL, AND BY NO MEANS BRIGHT.

an appropriate response from cartoonists.

The work of the vaccine board, begun by Dr Pearson, soon foundered because the sponsors withdrew, and also because of Jenner's open anxiety about safety standards. The second vaccination institution, the Royal Jennerian Society, got off to a good start with financial support from the public and the promise of support by Jenner, writing from Berkeley. Premises were found and a resident vaccinator, Dr Walker, appointed.

Dr Walker, who had pioneered Jenner's work in the Mediterranean, was an eccentric and rather forbidding character, and unfortunately there was a clash of personalities between him and Jenner. Later he resigned but went on doing useful work on his own in the London Vaccine Institute, and the Royal Jennerian Society gradually faded out.

Eventually parliament voted £3,000 running costs for a vaccination institute under the direction of the Royal College of Physicians. Jenner was not a member of the College and seemed to be excluded, but was then made Director. When he nominated eight vaccinators from Gloucestershire, seven were rejected by the board, and Jenner resigned angrily. However, James Moore, brother of Sir John Moore of Corunna, a loyal supporter and able administrator appeared. Moore kept in contact with Jenner who was able to give advice about keeping up standards and about developing the technique of vaccination.

Jenner was lucky to win the personal interest of the Royal Family and of the Court. King George III permitted Jenner to dedicate to him the second edition of *The Inquiry*, dated 1800. Jenner was appointed Physician Extraordinary to King George IV in 1821.

In time Jenner found himself in financial difficulties. He had been encouraged to live and practise in London, but he found that in furthering vaccination he had sacrificed his name as a physician and surgeon; he was only being used as a vaccinator. The King appreciated his position and recommended a petition which Jenner had drawn up to the House of Commons for the award of a Treasury grant. The House thereupon commissioned an enquiry to find out whether vaccination was in fact a boon to humanity, whether Jenner had discovered the method, and how much money he had made out of it.

The anti-Jenner lobby produced witnesses who did not stand up to cross-examination, and they tried to show that Jenner could not claim that the discovery was original. Indeed, a Farmer Jesty from Dorset had inoculated his own family with cow pox in 1774, but had done no more.

It was hard for the House of Commons Committee to work out how much Jenner should receive. If, for example, it was considered that he should be paid a royalty of ten shillings for every life saved per year he would be entitled to £20,000 per annum! A lump sum was decided upon. The country was at war, funds were limited and, by a majority of three, Jenner was awarded £10,000.

Jenner had to wait two years for his money, and when it did come the taxman had already deducted £1,000! Within a few years, however, a committee of the College of Physicians advised the Government how effective vaccination was, and the House debated another grant of £10,000. At the last minute the member for Newport proposed an amendment that the sum be doubled, so Jenner received £20,000 (this time tax free). But by now Catherine was ill and the Jenners had already returned to Berkeley and Cheltenham. Jenner resumed practice and, assisted by his nephew, offered to vaccinate everybody who wished to come to him.

A legion of supporters and vaccine missionaries emerged during these ten years. Dr John Lettsom, was one of the most able and influential physicians

Overleaf After the opposition to vaccination was proved wrong, it became quite fashionable to be inoculated. Many doctors set up in business to do little else but this.

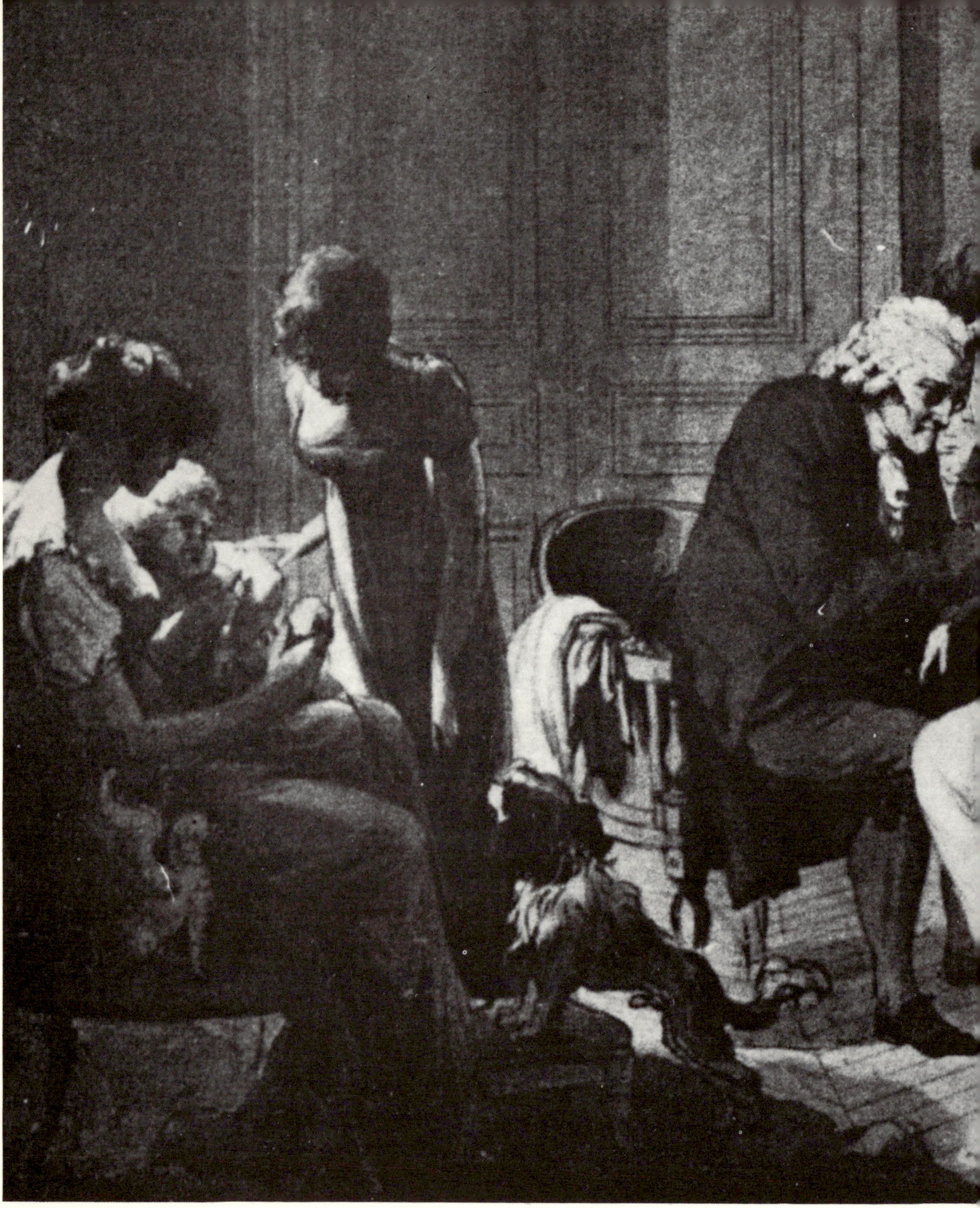

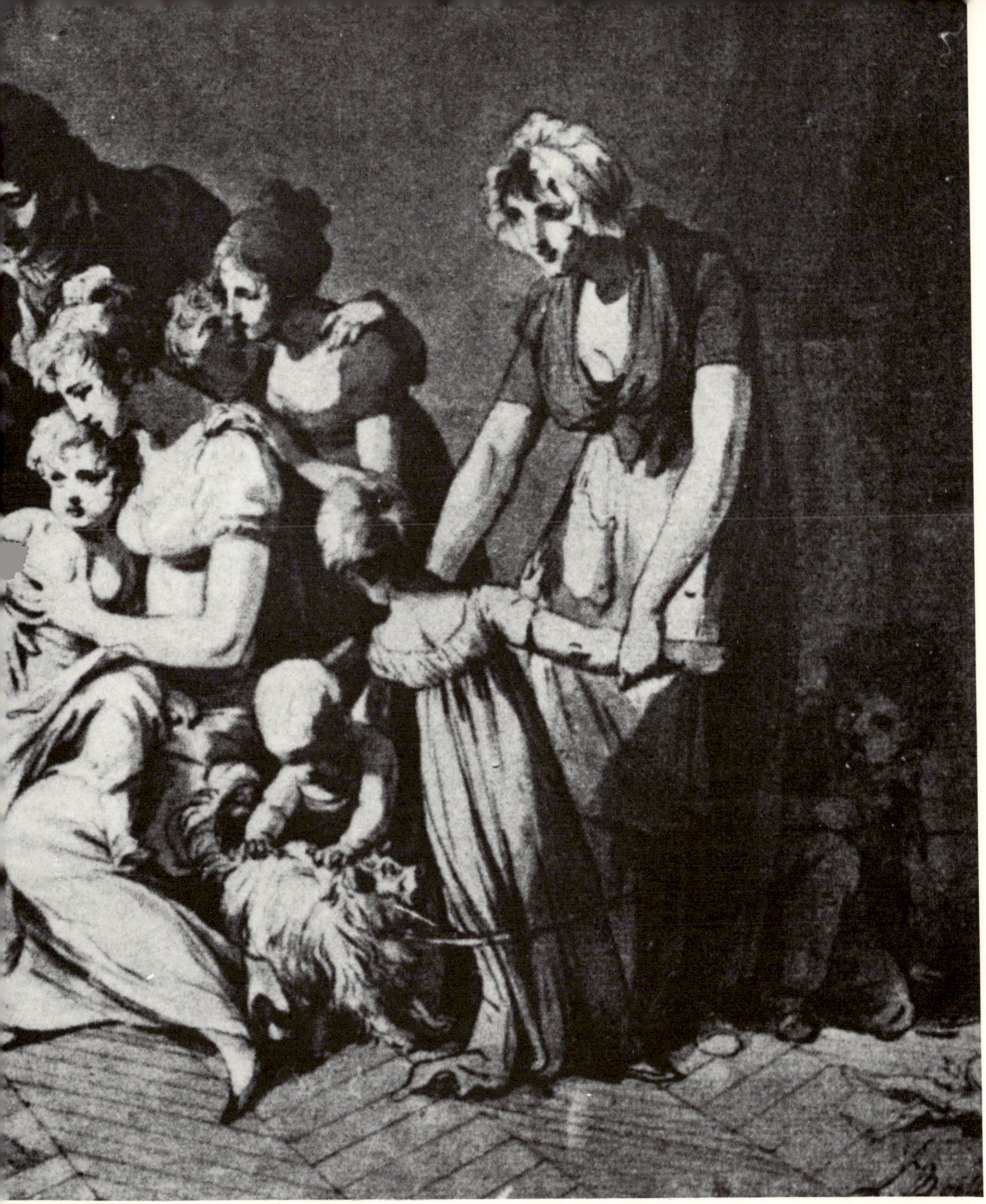

of the time and also a statistician. During the first parliamentary enquiry he was asked: "Do you think that the inoculation of the smallpox has lessened the deaths occasioned by smallpox?" His answer was "No! I think it has increased the number of deaths by extending the disease . . . 36,000 of our fellow subjects are annually sacrificed by the smallpox. *But out of 60,000 vaccinated only three have died, and they not of the smallpox.*"

Another early friend was Mr William Fermore who also found that people who milked cows could be immune from smallpox. He sensibly sought Jenner's advice when vaccination did not take, so George Jenner took lymph to Oxfordshire and vaccinated 326 people—176 of these were successfully tested with smallpox.

In July 1801 Dr Marshall and Dr Walker were sent by the Government to vaccinate the fleet and garrison in the Mediterranean from Gibraltar to Egypt. They halted one smallpox epidemic in Minorca. A Jennerian Institute was set up at Malta, where the Governor said that Dr Marshall "rendered the most essential service to the inhabitants by the introduction of vaccine inoculation, by which the ravages of the smallpox, so dreadful in this climate, were prevented." Dr Walker accompanied and made a great contribution to the military expedition to Egypt by vaccinating the army and navy, and Napoleon was quick to realize the health advantage that the British Forces had over his. (One hundred and forty years later the health of the British troops in Egypt played a part in the victory of El Alamein over German and Italian troops afflicted by dysentry). It was the same Dr Walker, rather gruff in manner and eccentric, who later clashed with Jenner over the management of the affairs of the Royal Jennerian Society.

Besides the gold medal of the London Medical Society, which Dr Lettsom received on his behalf,

Jenner was honoured in Britain by the Navy with a medal, the Physical Society of Guy's Hospital, the Medical Societies of Edinburgh and Manchester, The Royal Humane Society, the University of Oxford (with a testimonial and later, an Honorary M.D.) and the Royal College of Physicians of Edinburgh. He was awarded the freedom of the cities of London, Edinburgh, Liverpool, Glasgow and Dublin, and of the Burgh of Kirkaldy. Perhaps the best testimonial came through a surgeon friend, Richard Dunning and the Medical Society of Plymouth who commissioned James Northcote to paint Jenner's portrait. It is said that Jenner preferred this portrait to any of the others.

But Dunning of Plymouth did something else for Jenner and posterity, he introduced a new word into the English language—vaccination.

8 *World Opinion, Past and Present*

"Jenner, Ah, we can refuse nothing to that man." With these words the Emperor Napoleon summarized the gratitude of France and indeed the whole world to Jenner's vaccination and the consequent prevention of smallpox. It has been remarked wryly that the greatest testimony to Napoleon was his recognition of the benefits of vaccination and his willingness to acknowledge the great contribution made to humanity by a native of an enemy country.

Napoleon's remark about Jenner is said to be the result of a letter addressed by Jenner to the Emperor to request the release of a friend:

> "Sire,
>
> "Having by the blessings of Providence, made a discovery of which all nations acknowledge the beneficial effects, I presume upon that plea alone, with great deference, to request a favour from your Imperial Majesty, who early appreciated the importance of vaccination, and encouraged its propagation, and who is universally admitted to be a patron of the arts.
>
> "My humble request is that your Imperial Majesty will graciously permit two of my friends, both men of science and literature, to return to England; one, Mr. William Thomas Williams, residing at Nancy; the other Dr Wickham, at present in Geneva. Should your Imperial Majesty be pleased to listen to the prayer of my petition, you will impress my mind with sentiments never to be effaced.
>
> "I have the honour to be, with most profound deference and respect, Your Imperial Majesty's most obedient and humble servant,
>
> Edward Jenner"

Emperor Napoleon Bonaparte was quick to realise the importance of Jenner's work. He had the French troops inoculated to boost their morale and improve their health in the wars against the British.

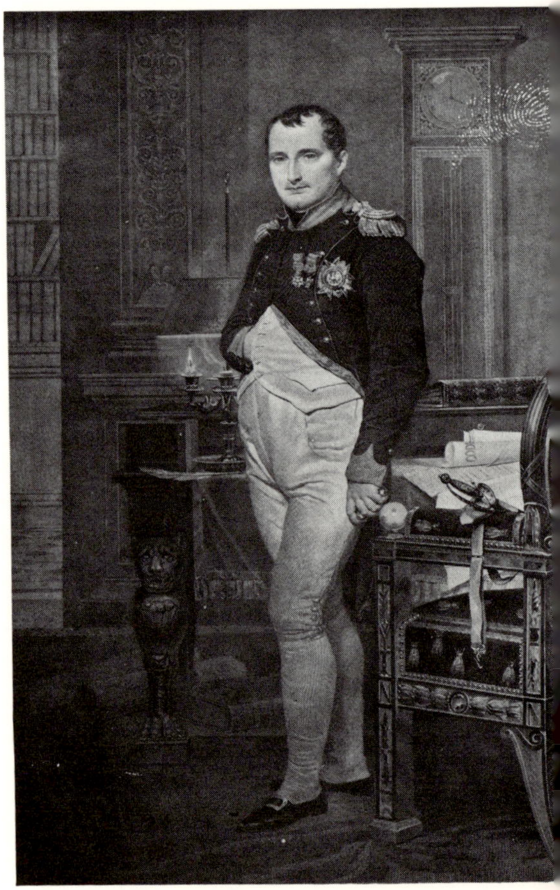

Napoleon and Josephine were waiting at Nancy for a change of horses for their chariot. Mr Williams was in the crowd and seized his opportunity to present the letter but he was held back by the guards. Josephine heard the name Jenner and is reputed to have said, "But Sire, this letter comes from Dr Jenner," and then Napoleon gave his historic reply. However, Jenner's request was not granted until the following year, when Napoleon was handed a duplicate copy of the letter by his physician.

Jenner's reputation on the Continent was so great that several people were released as a result of his personal appeals, and certificates declaring immunity from arrest were also written which stated "The holder is a patient of Dr Jenner and this journey is necessary for his/her health." Jenner also obtained the release of a vaccinator imprisoned by the King of Spain on a piracy charge.

Napoleon sent Dr Aubert to England in 1801 to secure all the information he could about vaccination and to open a vaccine institute in Paris. It was imperial policy to boost the morale of the French troops by any efforts to reduce illness and the effects of wounding. Napoleon was ably supported by his chief surgeon Baron Larrey.

Perhaps the greatest ambassador for vaccination amongst the countries of Europe was a Swiss doctor who qualified in Edinburgh and practiced in Vienna, Dr de Carro. Curiously enough vaccination had reached him from Dr Pearson's dubious vaccine institute, but de Carro soon contacted Jenner because he had some failures with the Pearson lymph. He was sure that vaccination was the answer to the smallpox problem but was unable to obtain any local supplies. In spite of the war, Jenner sent him lymph through the British Legation in Vienna. It survived the journey and enabled de Carro to develop and spread the practice throughout the whole of Europe and to Russia. De Carro, with the help of Lord Elgin, was largely responsible for bringing vaccination to India, Italy, Greece and Turkey as well as Baghdad.

After a false start the King of Spain introduced vaccination to the Spanish possessions in America by a three year, and highly successful, expedition. Sailing from Corunna, the activity of the cow pox was maintained by a succession of vaccinations of the twenty-six unvaccinated children aboard. At Puerto Rico one section of the expedition headed south for Buenos Aires, and the other reached Havanna and Mexico. Within three years vaccination had reached the Philippine Islands and China.

Jenner had, of course, successfully sent good lymph to Newfoundland but it was through Dr Lettsom that cow pox vaccination reached the U.S.A. He obtained fresh active lymph from the vaccine institute in Bath and managed to get it to a colleague in Massachusetts, who promptly vaccinated six of his seven children and then publicly inoculated one of them with smallpox, a dramatic and effective advertisement. However, smallpox inoculation had previously been introduced, not without public disturbance, in 1721 at the suggestion of Cotton Mather. Unfortunately in the wild enthusiasm cow pox became mixed up with the smallpox used earlier. Once again the new method failed because of lack of attention to detail. Presidents Adams and Jefferson intervened and saved vaccination by obtaining a fresh supply of clean lymph. Jefferson took on the work himself, and successfully vaccinated his own children, his family, relations and neighbours. He also began to vaccinate the North American Indians.

Gradually reports of the effect of vaccination on the incidence and mortality of smallpox began to come in. In Denmark 9,728 people died from smallpox between 1762 and 1792. Vaccination

President John Adams of America realised that failures of early inoculations in America were due to carelessness over handling the materials. This prevented inoculation falling into disrepute.

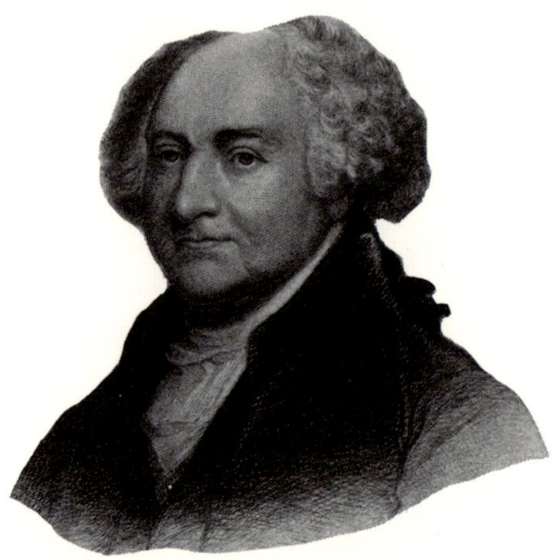

began in 1802. Smallpox inoculation was abolished in 1810. Between 1810 and 1819 not a single case of smallpox occurred.

In other places, too, the story was one of success. In Havana, where smallpox had been rife, there was no death for two years. In Spanish America "small pox [was] extinguished."

In France, 2,671,602 persons were vaccinated, and only seven cases of smallpox occurred in these. In India, 243,175 persons were vaccinated and there was not a single case of smallpox in Bombay for two years. In Italy, Dr Sacco reported 60,000 vaccinations by 1802. And in Germany smallpox was now almost unknown after an efficient vaccination policy.

Russia's chief of the civil medical department was Dr Alexander Crichton, physician to the Westminster Hospital, later to become Sir Alexander Crichton. On 12th September 1812 he wrote from St. Petersburg (now Leningrad):

> "Dear Sir,
>
> "The re-establishment of peace between England and Russia being happily concluded, I embrace an early opportunity of sending you a letter on the state of vaccination in this empire . .
>
> "The whole number of children vaccinated in the Empire amounts to 1,235,597. Now supposing according to a well-founded rule of calculation, that before the introduction of vaccination, every seventh child died, annually, of smallpox, vaccination has saved the lives of 176,154 children in this Empire."

The Russian Emperor was so enthusiastic about vaccination that he ordered the vaccination of the whole Empire in three years, the establishment of vaccination committees in every town and included the injunction that the practice be introduced into all schools and that students be taught to practice it.

And with the results came the letters of acclaim,

the decorations and the presents. The National Institute of France elected him an Associate Member—a high honour. He was congratulated personally by the Emperor of Russia, the King of Germany and Blücher. In Germany, for many years a national festival was held on May 14th, the anniversary of the day Jenner vaccinated James Phipps. A letter of congratulations from Germany informed Jenner that he had received the Diploma of the Royal Academy of Science, while from East Germany news came of a monument erected to him "and Heaven may conserve your life to the most remote time." The Royal Society of Göttingen made him an honorary member, as did the Royal Economical Society of Madrid.

He was awarded the degree of Ll.D. by the Harvard University in Massachusetts, and an honour from the American Philosophical Society was signed by Thomas Jefferson. The New Hampshire Society sent him a diploma. Calcutta sent £3,000, Bombay £2,000 and Madras £1,383. Other honours flooded in. The Dowager Empress of Russia sent a valuable diamond ring. Jenner declined a Russian decoration on the grounds that his means were inadequate to support it.

The most touching of all the tributes came from ten chiefs of North American Indian tribes. Jenner had forwarded details about vaccination and the necessary instructions to the Chiefs. Their gift to Jenner of Wampum, cowrie shells sewn into a belt or on a string, was regarded by them as a pact of the highest token of friendship. Their message was marked by the respective signs of their tribes.

"Brother,

"Our father—[Governor of Canada] has delivered to us the book you sent to instruct us how to use the discovery which the Great Spirit made to you, whereby the smallpox, that fatal enemy of our tribes, may be driven from the

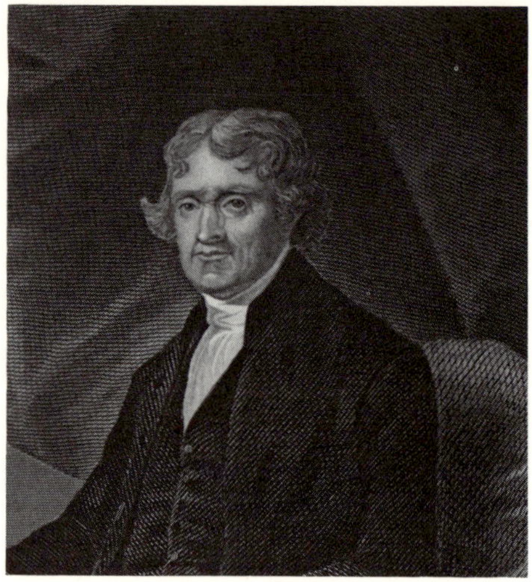

President Jefferson of America was also an enthusiastic supporter of Jenner's work. He had all his family inoculated and introduced vaccination to the North American Indians.

earth. We have deposited your book in the hands of the men of skill our father employs to attend us when sick or wounded. We shall not fail to teach our children to speak the name of Jenner, and to thank the Great Spirit for bestowing upon him so much wisdom and so much benevolence.

"We send with this a belt and a string of wampum, in token of our acceptance of your precious gift, and we beseech the Great Spirit to take care of you in this world and in the land of spirits."

Edward Jenner lived at a time of revolutions in political, industrial and scientific fields. He contributed significantly to the Scientific Revolution by his work in chemistry and natural history. His contribution to medical science, cow pox vaccination, stood as a revolution on its own. The only previous breakthrough in medical science to compare with it was the discovery of the circulation of the blood by William Harvey in 1628 and the world was to wait for another revolutionary idea until 1846 and 1867, respectively the discovery of anaesthesia, and the birth of modern surgery through Lister's publication of his work on antisepsis.

Jenner's work on cow pox and vaccination significantly reduced the sum of human suffering. It is a mistake to believe that Jenner's contribution to humanity should only be viewed in the light of the smallpox threat of those days. The world had to fall back on Jenner during the nineteenth century and, today, nearly two hundred years later, the menace of smallpox still lurks in corners of the world and an efficient worldwide vaccination policy is still essential. As recently as March, 1973, the two deaths in London during a threatened outbreak highlighted the dangers which still exist.

It was not long after Jenner's death that the impetus of vaccination lessened and technical atten-

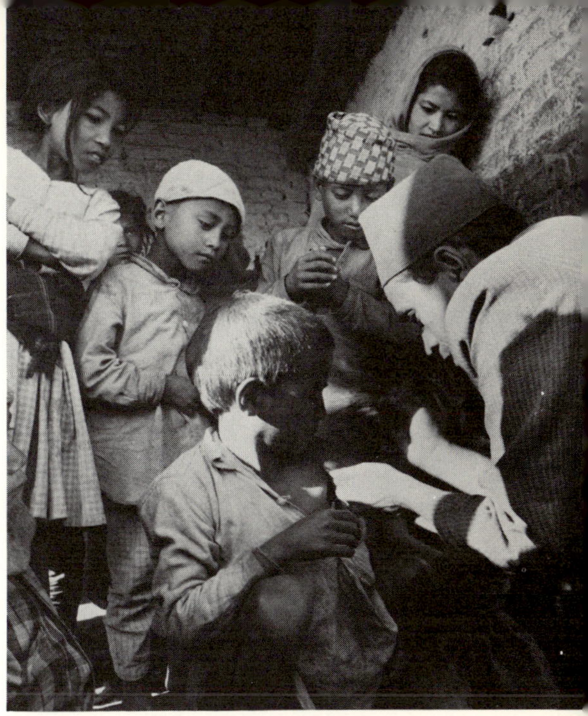

Above A health worker inoculates the children of a Nepalese village as part of a programme to stamp out smallpox in Nepal.

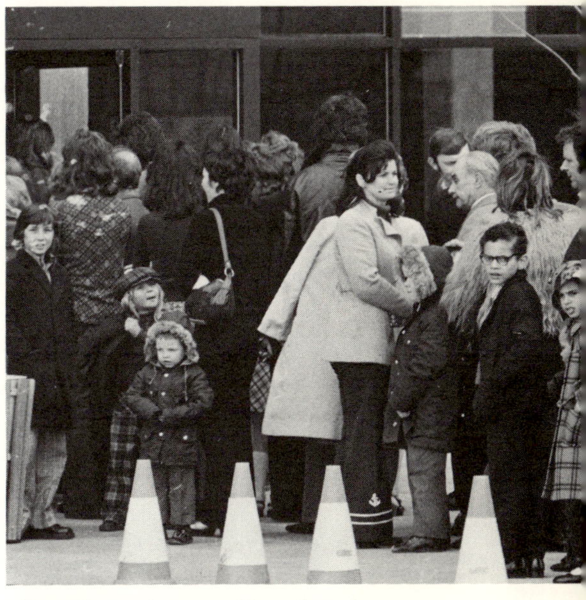

Above Queueing outside a London health centre for smallpox vaccinations in April 1973, after an outbreak of the disease in the city.

tion to detail slackened. Severe epidemics occurred in Italy in 1853, in England in 1864, and in Australia and the United States in 1884. The cry was "back to Jenner" and republication of his *Inquiry* was called for. The Germans, however, kept up vaccination as did the Japanese, and remained free of epidemics.

More recently, a grim reminder of this vicious disease occurred at Christmas, 1961, when five Pakistani immigrants entered England. They were said to have had valid certificates of vaccination, but they all had smallpox, and two of them died. Immediately a bushfire type of spread occurred among the contacts and by the time the epidemic was brought under control 62 cases had occurred and 24 people had died, including two doctors. It was reported that of those affected, 40 were hospital staff who had neglected vaccination. Even in 1972 and 1973 an outbreak was reported in Bangladesh affecting between twelve and thirteen thousand people.

Only a few years ago smallpox was known to be present (endemic) in forty-six countries. Today four countries continue to struggle with a hard core of the disease: India, Pakistan, Bangladesh and Ethiopia. Modern air travel increases the chances of the virus being spread around the world at any moment. Effective control still depends upon the maintenance of high standards of vaccination and in scrupulous care in the preservation and usage of the lymph. Jenner and Moore vaccinated four areas of skin. Today only one site is used, but frequent revaccination becomes mandatory. In an outbreak of smallpox—vaccination, the key to the control of the situation—is backed up by the exhaustive tracing of contacts and their isolation and quarantine.

Modern vaccination with vaccinia virus is rarely followed by complications, but encephalitis (inflammation of the brain) occurs about five times in

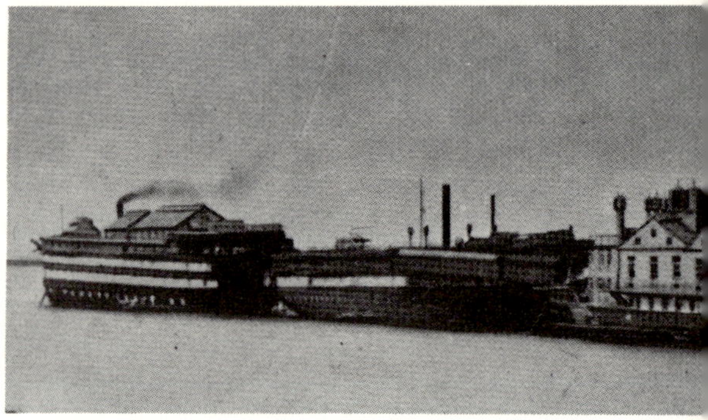

Hospital ships on the Thames near London were used to isolate patients suffering from smallpox during outbreaks of the disease in 1900.

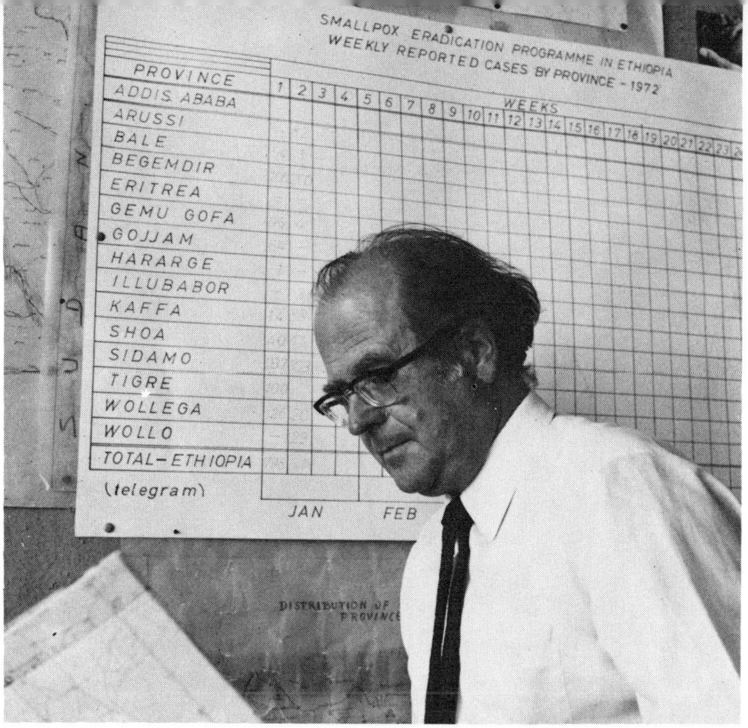

Left A World Health Organisation scientist checks the progress of the smallpox eradication programme in Ethiopia.

Below Fast, easy modern ways of travelling increase the risk of smallpox spreading across the world. In 1963 alone, as the map shows, smallpox travelled by air from south-east Asia to Sweden, from India to Poland and from central Africa to Switzerland. From Calcutta a smallpox carrier went by boat to Suez, but the health authorities took precautions, and prevented the disease reaching the Mediterranean region.

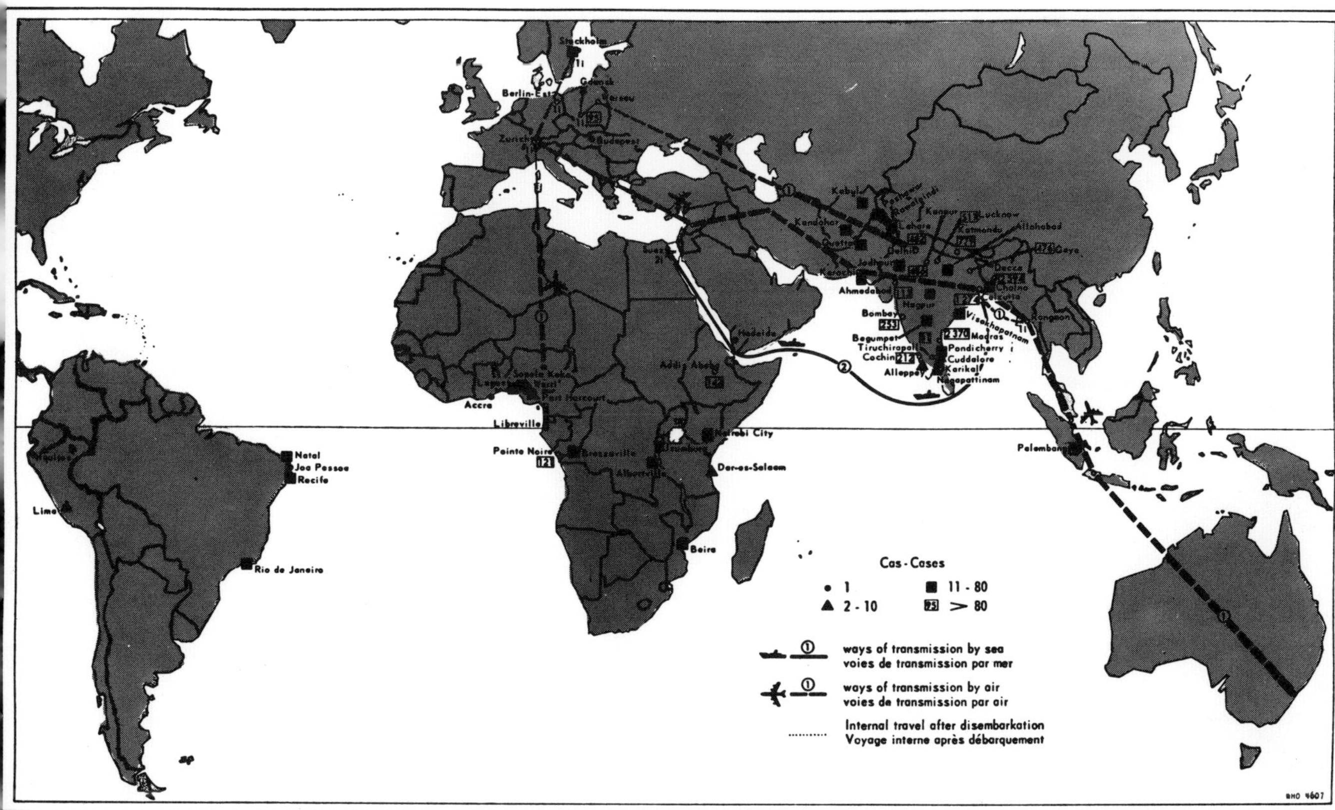

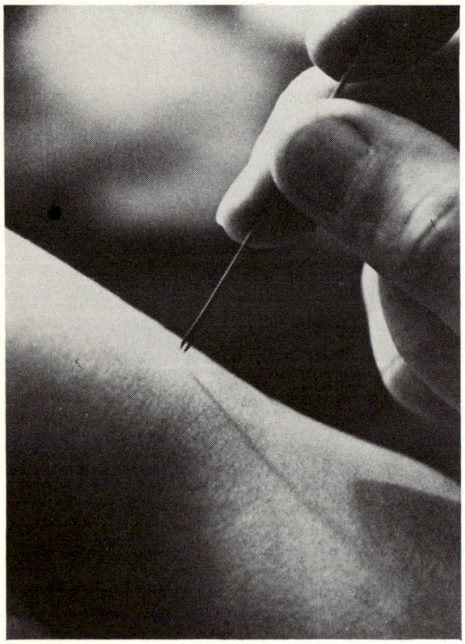

Above A bifurcated (two pronged) needle used in many smallpox eradication programmes. The needle is dipped in the vaccine and the skin is pricked very quickly about fifteen times. This method is quick and effective.

Below A very modern vaccine jet injector. The bottle containing the vaccine is above the "barrel" of the injector. This is a far cry from the early, primitive instruments from China and India.

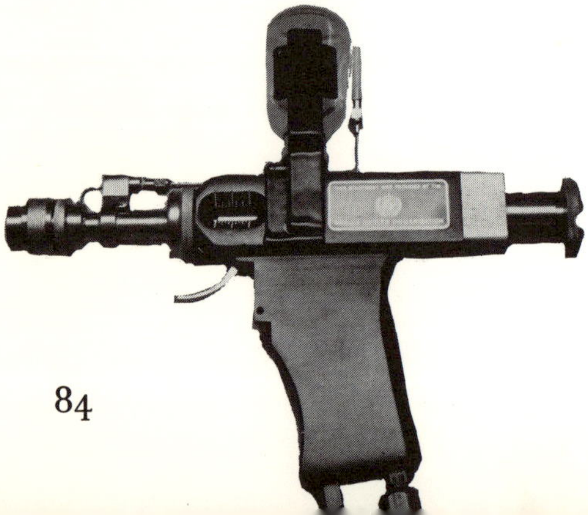

a million cases and a generalized infection can also occur.

Jenner's work has some meaning in the development of another aspect of preventive medicine. Louis Pasteur must surely have been influenced by the story of vaccination, and, having shown that diseases could be carried by bacterial infection, developed solutions containing bacteria modified or weakened by heat or alcohol, which he called "vaccines" in memory of Jenner. These vaccines caused a mild subclinical attack of the relevant disease (like cow pox) and yet gave acquired active immunity. By his vaccines Pasteur restored the fortunes of France after the Franco–Prussian war of 1870 by controlling the devastation of sheep and cattle caused by anthrax, and by saving the crippled silkworm industry from silkworm infection. The serious problem of rabies was also controlled by a vaccine.

In this century, there has been a big development of vaccines and similar immunity-producing modifications of bacterial products (e.g. formol toxoids). For example, in 1953 Salk made a vaccine by growing poliomyelitis virus on monkey kidneys and killing the virus by adding formaldehyde. Sabin followed in 1955 with a live but greatly attenuated virus. A vaccine against tuberculosis was developed in 1906 by Calmette and Guérin (B.C.G.). The bovine strain of tuberculosis was attenuated by being grown for several years on a potato medium and by being inhibited by bile-salts. After a period of success, Jenner's old warning about attention to detail became a reality when at Lübeck in 1930 a batch of the vaccine contained live virulent tubercle bacilli and seventy-two out of 251 children died. This incident put back the adoption of B.C.G. by the United Kingdom for many years. This was the sort of disaster, which Jenner's opponents, Woodville and Pearson might have caused, and which

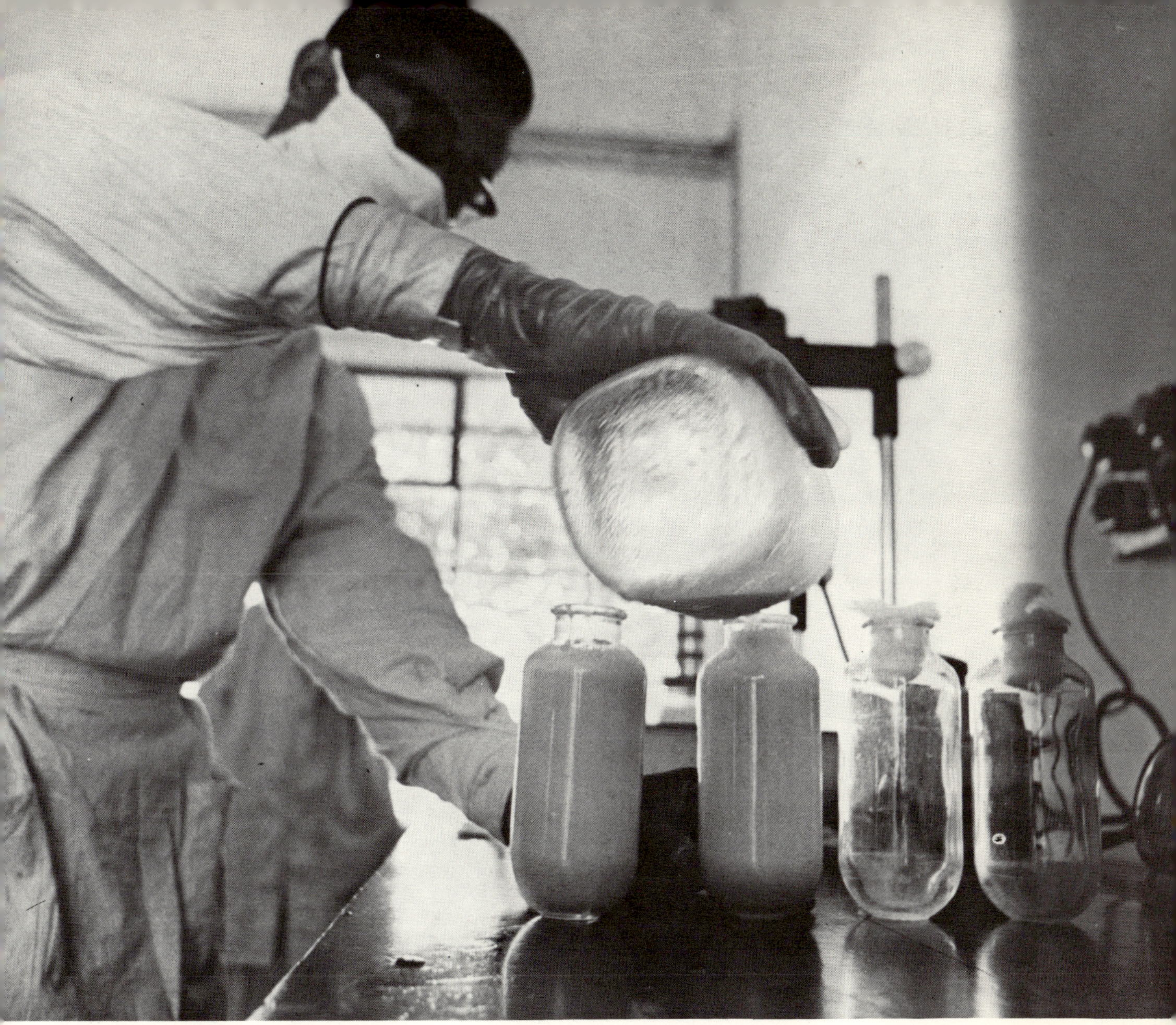

Processing crude lymph during the manufacture of anti-smallpox vaccine.

Jenner feared; it could have defeated all his efforts to establish vaccination against smallpox.

Jenner realized that in some cases immunity was not always long-lasting. Today this fact is fully appreciated and is the reason why revaccination or "booster" doses of vaccine are given in certain circumstances. Another phenomenon first reported by Jenner and well known today was hypersensitivity

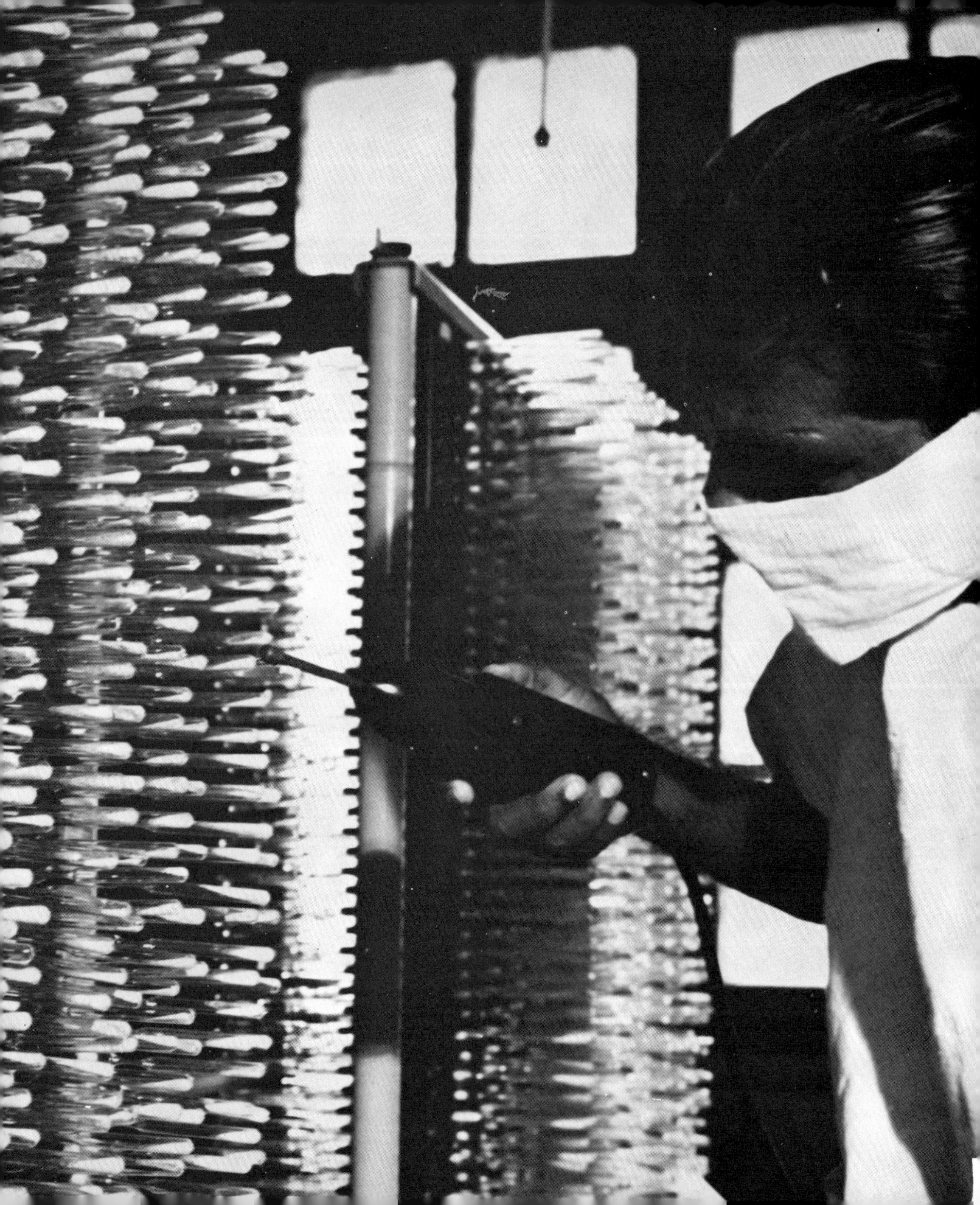

following vaccination—in other words a form of allergy.

It has already been mentioned that Jenner was impressed by the possible association of the cow pox of those days with a pustular condition of horses' heels called grease. He was the first person to realize relationships in infective diseases. Today, several types of pox virus affecting different species of animals are recognized.

We encounter many instances today when we are reminded of Jenner. It may be when we receive a vaccination for travel abroad, or when we hear of a smallpox epidemic, and perhaps see a harrassed medical officer of health on television explaining how an outbreak can be contained. We may also remember Jenner when we consider the heat of a candle flame, the dangers of exposure in the snow, the free flight of a balloon, the wormcasts on the lawn—even when the house martins return to the eaves and we hear the first cuckoo in spring.

Opposite and below The weapon with which smallpox is now fought throughout the world—powdery freeze-dried vaccine which remains at the peak of its effectiveness wherever it is used. A weapon first discovered by an observant English country doctor.

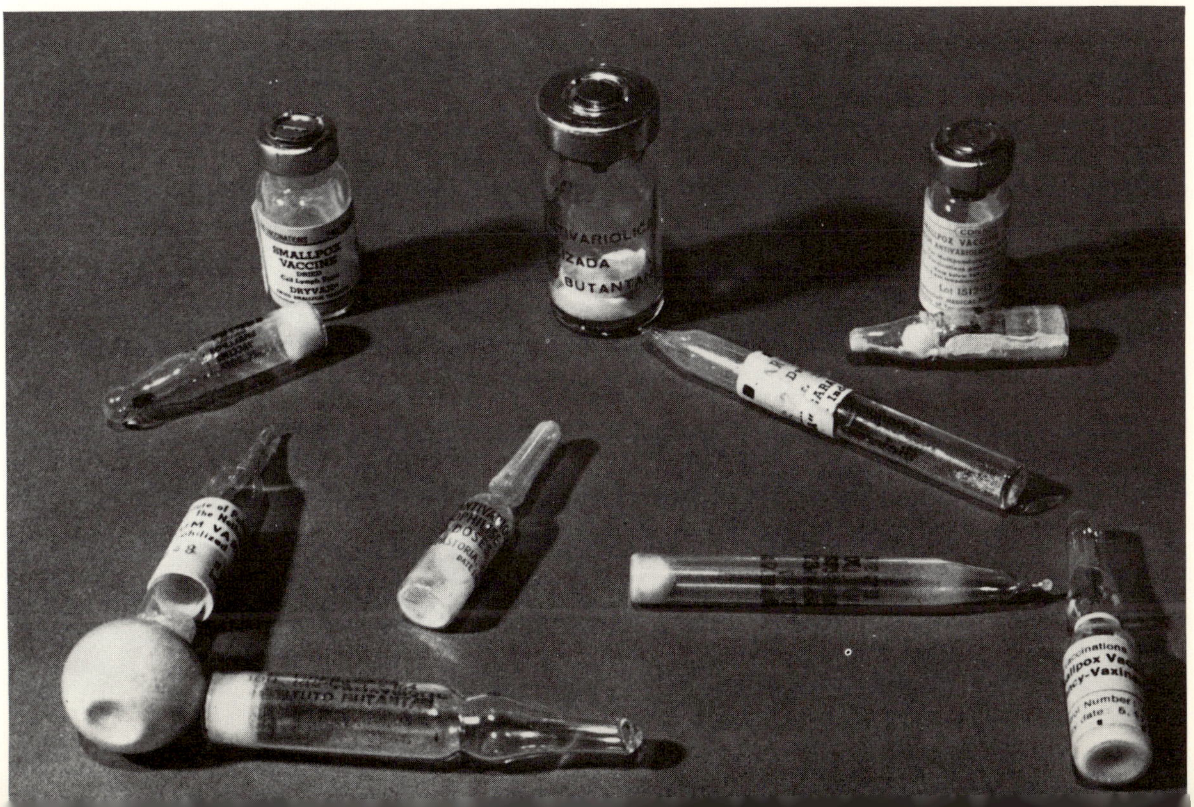

Date Chart

1749	(17th May) Edward Jenner is born
1754	His parents die
1757	He goes to school at Wootton-under-Edge and Cirencester
1761	Is apprenticed to Mr Ludlow—surgeon of Chipping Sodbury
1770	Becomes a pupil of the surgeon-scientist John Hunter, London and attends the Windmill School of Anatomy. Obtains certificates in medical studies
1773	Returns to Berkeley, Gloucestershire and begins practice as country surgeon
1775	Assists Hunter with the study of hibernation of hedgehogs. Hunter sends his immortal letter, "But why think, why not try the experiment." Begins to study the migration of birds.
1778	Describes disease of the coronary arteries
1783	Is involved in an early unmanned balloon ascent
1784	Purifies antimony tartrate by recrystallization
1786	Gives an account of exposure and frostbite in a blizzard
1787	Discovers the behaviour of the young cuckoo in the nest
1787	His paper on the cuckoo is submitted to the Royal Society
1788	(6th March) Edward Jenner marries Catherine Kingscote
1789	Elected F.R.S.
1793	John Hunter dies of a heart disease described by Jenner
1795	Jenner nearly dies of typhus

1796	Jenner decides to "try the experiment" of inoculating James Phipps (aged 8) with the cowpox from a milkmaid, Sarah Nelmes
1796	(19th July) James Phipps pronounced immune from smallpox
1798	Jenner publishes his first paper (*An Inquiry*) on vaccination. Cowpox vaccination first successful in London
1801	The Royal Navy Mediterranean fleet vaccinated. Success in batttles with Napoleon
1801	Napoleon sends a doctor to England to learn vaccination and adopts it for all his armed forces
1801	Thomas Jefferson, President of the U.S.A. vaccinates his own family, relations and the North American Indians
1802	Vaccination established in Europe and over much of the rest of the world.
1802	First Parliamentary enquiry into vaccination and grant to Jenner of £10,000.
1805	Jenner writes to Napoleon with a successful request for the release of detainees
1806	Second Parliamentary enquiry and grant of £20,000
1812	Over $1\frac{1}{4}$ million people vaccinated in Russia. Vaccination taught in Russian schools by order of the Emperor
1815	Death of Mrs Jenner. Jenner returns to his work on the migration of birds
1820	Jenner has a stroke
1821	He is appointed Physician extraordinary to King George IV
1823	(24th January) Jenner dies
1824	Posthumous publication *On the Migration of Birds*

Glossary

ALLERGY Sensitivity of the body to other substances, usually food or bacterial proteins

ANGINA PECTORIS A symptom of disease in the coronary arteries of the heart

ANILENE DYE A coloured derivative of anilene used for staining bacteria

ANTHRAX A contagious and mortal infection of sheep and cattle which can affect humans

ARTERIOSCLEROSIS Hardening and degeneration of the arteries related to ageing and excessive cigarette smoking and sugar intake

ATTENUATION Weakening the virulence of germs by repeated subculture. The weakened germs, however, remain capable of stimulating immunity.

AXILLA The armpit, which contains lymph nodes

BILLS OF MORTALITY A way of publishing the causes of death throughout the kingdom—nowadays called the Registrar General's returns

BOOSTER Succeeding injections of vaccines or revaccination to boost immunity

CONTAGIOUS DISEASE A disease spread by contact from one person to another or by droplets or by fomites (see below)

CORONARY ARTERIES The arteries which supply blood to the heart muscle

COW POX Disease of cows caused by a pox virus spreading to humans by contact

CUTIS The skin

DEGENERATION The chemical changes associated with the wearing out and reduction of function of the tissues and organs of the body

DROPLET SPREAD Spread of disease by fine droplets from the mouth during speech, coughing and sneezing

DONOR One who gives to another. In the medical sense, for example, a blood donor, a kidney donor

ELECTRON MICROSCOPE A microscope using a stream of electrons instead of light to show up minute detail

ENDEMIC DISEASES A disease which occurs in a particular locality

FOMITES Any object, for example clothes and bedding, by which a contagious disease can be spread

FORMOL TOXOID Toxin (poisons) of bacteria treated by the chemical formaldehyde but still capable of stimulating immunity

FROSTBITE Burning (coagulation) of the skin caused by intense cold

F.R.S. Fellow of the Royal Society of London

HYPERSENSITIVITY Extremely sensitive form of allergy, for example to certain kinds of food

HYPOTHESIS A supposition based on a reasoned argument to be proved or disproved by facts or experiment

IMMUNITY Protection against infections, the result of having had a particular disease following inoculation with a vaccine (acquired immunity). Babies have some temporary immunity derived from their mothers (natural immunity)

INFECTION Invasion of the body by bacteria and viruses

INFLAMMATION The reaction of the living body to injury, infection and infestation by parasites. Usually manifest by redness, pain, swelling, local heat and loss of function

INOCULATION Injection of a vaccine to stimulate immunity to a particular disease

INSOMNIA Inability to sleep

LYMPH The watery alkaline fluid from the tissues of the body which finds its way back into the circulation via the lymphatic vessels. Also the term used to describe the fluid matter in the cowpox vesicle (blister) which contained the cowpox virus and was used for vaccination

NEURITIS Inflammation of the nerves

NITROUS OXIDE (N_2O) Laughing gas, used as an anaesthetic

ORGANISM A living thing—usually referring to bacteria

PARALYSIS Complete loss of function of muscles

PASSAGE Passing an infection from one animal to another which may increase virulence

PLAGUE A mortal infection caused by the bacteria *Pasteurella pestis* transmitted by rats and fleas; The Black Death

POLIOMYELITIS An acute virus infection of the nervous system causing paralysis of muscles—infantile paralysis

POSTMORTEM Dissection of the body after death, to find the cause of death

PUSTULE A small blister containing pus and infective matter

QUARANTINE Isolation or segregation of persons or animals likely to be infected with a contagious disease

QUILL Literally the quill of a feather—in which cowpox lymph was transported in Jenner's days

RABIES Hydrophobia, a form of madness of dogs, caused by a virus, and transmissable to humans

SCAR The permanent marking of the skin following injury, operation or infection

SMALLPOX Acute, very contagious and deadly disease caused by the pox virus, variola

STROKE Temporary or permanent paralysis, caused by a stoppage of blood, to, or bleeding into, the brain

TUBERCLE BACILLUS The bacteria which causes tuberculosis

TYPHOID An acute severe disease spread by water

and contaminated food

TYPHUS An acute mortal disease spread by lice and fleas and rats

ULCER Any breach in a surface of the body; for example, the skin

VACCINATION The word coined by Mr Dunning, Plymouth surgeon, to describe Jenner's cowpox inoculation, and used today for any injection employed to produce immunity to a particular disease

VACCINE A suspension of weakened (attentuated) or killed bacteria which if injected will stimulate immunity to a particular disease

VACCINIA The pox virus developed from cowpox and now used for vaccination against smallpox

VARICELLA Chicken pox

VARIOLA VACCINAE Cowpox

VARIOLA Smallpox

VESICLE Small blister containing serum

VIRAEMIA The presence of a virus in the blood

VIRULENCE The strength of a bacteria or virus in producing disease

VIRUS Originally meaning a venom or poison, but adopted to mean an ultramicroscopic and bacterial filter-passing organism

Further Reading

There are two major sources of information about Jenner—his life and his work. Dr John Baron, the official biographer, was personally associated with Jenner in his later years, and through him Jenner comes alive. Mr Le Fanu, formerly Librarian of the Royal College of Surgeons of England, compiled and assembled a bibliography in a work of great assistance to all who would study Jenner. The following list comprises a short bibliography which may be helpful

Baron, John, *The Life of Edward Jenner,* M.D., LL.D., F.R.S., in two volumes (1827)

Le Fanu, W. R., *A Bibliography of Edward Jenner 1749–1823,* (Harvey and Blythe, London, 1951)

Drewitt, F. D., *The Life of Edward Jenner,* M.D., F.R.S. (Longmans, London, 1931)

——, *The Notebook of Edward Jenner* (Oxford University Press, London, 1931)

Fisk, Dorothy, *Dr Jenner of Berkeley* (Heinemann, London, 1959)

Bishop, W. J., *The Early History of Surgery* (Hale, London, 1960)

Haggard, H. W., *Devils, Drugs and Doctors* (Heinemann, London)

Turner, Grey, *The Hunterian Museum* (Cassell, London, 1946)

Dobson, Jessie, *John Hunter* (E. & S. Livingstone, London, 1969)

Churchill, Winston S., *The History of the English Speaking Peoples* (Cassell, London)

Fosbroke, T. D., *The Berkeley Manuscripts*

Index

Adams, U.S. President, 78
America, 78, 79, 80
Amyand, Claudius, 53
Antagonists, 54, 66, 71
Antimony tartrate, 25
Awards, financial, 71
—other, 74, 75, 80

Bagdad, 78
Balloon flight, 24
Bangladesh, 82
Banks, Joseph, 31
Barber Surgeons, 53
B.C.G., 84
Berkeley castle, 16
—fair, 16
—family, 21
—village of, 10–16, 64
Blizzard, 19
Blossom, cow, 64
Body snatchers, 28
Booster, 85

Canada, 80
Candle incident, 31
Carro, Dr. de, 77
Catherine the Great, 53
Chantry House, 19
Chicken pox, 45
Cline, Mr., 65
—letter to Jenner, 66
Clive, Robert, 22
Clubs, medical, 12
Coleridge, Samuel, 27
Contemporaries, 24–27
Coronary disease, 31
Cook, Captain, 22, 31
Cotton Mather, 78
Cotswolds, 16, 19
Counter irritation, 65
Cow Pox, Cline's case, 65
Cow Pox, definition, 57
—experiment, 59–64
Crichton, Sir Alexander, 79
Crystals, 25, 26
Cuckoo, 34–39

Dairymaids, 57–62
Davy, Sir Humphry, 25
Death of Jenner, 15
—of John Hunter, 32
Deaths from smallpox, 8, 45, 50, 54, 78–82
Deaths from smallpox inoculation, 54
Degrees, 30, 80
Denmark, 78
Dimsdale, Thomas, 53
Disease, coronary, 31
Dunning of Plymouth, 75

Earthworms, 39
Ehrlich, Paul, 55
Electron microscope, 41
Ethiopia, 82
Experiment, cowpox, 62
—cuckoos, 34–39
—hedgehogs, 33
—Hunter's letter, 33

Faraday, Michael, 25, 65
Flexner, Simon, 32
Fomites, 41
Fossils, 16
France, 24, 54, 76, 84
Freemartins, 34
Frostbite, 19
F.R.S., 24, 36

General Medical Council, 12
George I, 53
George III, 70
George IV, 70
Germany, 80, 82
Gradner, Edward—letter to, 62
Grease, Horses', 59
Greece, 78

Harvey, William, 81
Hedgehogs, 33
Hibernation, 33
Honours, 74–75
—abroad, 80
Horse Pox, 59, 60
House of Commons enquiry, 71
Hunter, John, 28
—collection of, 28
—death of, 32
—Jenner's friendship with, 12, 13, 28–32
—letters from, 13, 33, 34
—pupils of, 29, 65
—teaching by, 28, 32
Hunter, William, 28
Hypothermia, 19

India, 78–80
Indians, North American, 78, 80
Ingenhouse, Dr., 66
"Inquiry", 55, 64, 70, 82
Immunity, 60, 84, 85
Institute, Pneumatic, 25
—Vaccine, 70
Italy, 78, 79

Jackal, 34
Japan, 82
Jefferson, U.S. President 78, 80
Jenner, Edward
—apprenticed, 12
—awards to, 71, 80
—birth of, 10
—childhood, 11
—contemporaries of, 22–27
—death of, 15
—degrees awarded to, 30, 80
—description of, 10
—family of, 11, 12, 14
—inoculated with smallpox, 53
—marriage, 14
—poems of, 16, 27
—portrait, 75
—schooling, 11
Jenner, Mrs., 14
Jenner Museum, 21, 64
Josephine, Empress, 77

Laughing gas, 25
Lettsom, Dr., 57, 71, 74
Lister, Joseph, 55, 65, 81
London Vaccine Institute, 70
Louis XV, 45
Lubeck disaster, 84
Ludlow, Mr., 12

Malta, 74
Marshall, Dr., 74
Medical clubs, 12
—education, 32
Medical Society of London, 74

Medical Society of Plymouth, 75
Milkmaids, 57–62
Montagu, Lady Mary Wortley, 52
Moore, James, 70
Mortality, Bills of, 54, 57
Moseley, Dr., 68
Museum, Hunterian, 28, 31, 33
—Jenner, 21, 64

Napoleon, and Jenner's letter to, 76
Navy, 74
Nelmes, Sarah, 60
Northcote, James, 75
Nursery rhyme, 57

Pakistan, 82
Pasteur, Louis, 26, 55, 65, 84
Pearson, Dr., 68, 77
Phipps, James, 62, 64
Pneumatic Institute, Medical, 25
Poets, 25, 27
Pox virus, 41, 87

Raffles, Sir Stamford, 24
Registration, medical, 12
Revolutions, 24, 25
Royal College of Physicians, 30, 70, 71
Royal College of Surgeons, 30
Royal Commission, 54
Royal Jennerian Society, 70
Royal Society, 24, 36
Russia, 53, 78–80

Simpson, Sir James, 65
Smallpox, (Variola), 8, 41
—complications of, 45
—deaths from, 8, 45, 50, 54, 57, 78–82
—effects of, 45, 50
—effects of vaccination on, 78, 79
—inoculation, 50, 78, 79
—mortality (see deaths)
—recent outbreaks, 81, 82
—spread, 45, 54
Spain, 78, 80
Surgical training, 12, 32
Suttons, 53

Tartar emetic, 25
Temple of Vaccinia, 19
Thermometer, 33
Thesis, Content of a, 55
Training, surgical, 12, 32
Turkey, 78

U.S.A., 78, 80, 82
—Presidents of, 78, 80

Vaccination, beginnings, 66
—complications of, 82
—compulsory, 9
—effect of, 77, 82
—new word, 75
—Royal Commission on (1896), 54
—success of, 66, 74, 77, 81
—trouble with, 68, 78, 81
Vaccines, 84
Vaccine Board, 68–70
Varicella (Chicken pox), 45
Variola (see smallpox)
Variolation, 50, 54, 78, 79
Viraemia, 41
Viruses, 41

Walker, Dr., 70, 74
Wampum, 80
Watt, James, 24
Westwood, 41
Whale, 18, 34
Windmill, School of Anatomy, 28
Woodville, Dr., 68
World Health Organization, 9

Zoo (London), 24

Picture Credits

The author and publishers would like to thank all those who have given permission for copyright illustrations to appear on the following pages: Charing Cross Hospital Medical School, 40; J. E. Gethyn-Jones, 10, 18, 20, 21; the Jenner Trust, 13, 57 (bottom); the Mansell Collection, 8, 61; Mary Evans picture library, 16–17, 22 (top), 25, 26, 50, 56 (top), 69, 76, 78, 80; Paul Popper, 35, 36, 37; the Royal College of Surgeons, 11, 12, 22 (centre), 23, 28, 29, 58, 59, 63, 66–67; WHO, *frontispiece*, 9, 42–43, 44, 46–47, 48–49, 51, 52, 72–73, 81, 82, 83, 84, 85, 86, 87.